HORMONE THERAPY
AND THE BRAIN

*A clinical perspective
on the role of estrogen*

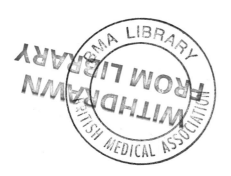

HORMONE THERAPY AND THE BRAIN

A clinical perspective on the role of estrogen

Victor W. Henderson, MD, MS

Kenneth and Bette Volk Professor of Neurology, and Professor of Gerontology and Psychology;
Chief of the Division of Cognitive Neuroscience and Neurogerontology;
University of Southern California, Los Angeles, California, USA

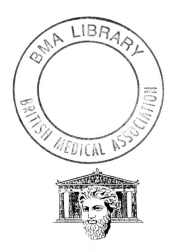

The Parthenon Publishing Group

International Publishers in Medicine, Science & Technology

NEW YORK   LONDON

Library of Congress Cataloging-in-Publication Data
Henderson, Victor W.
    Hormone therapy and the brain : a clinical
perspective on the role of estrogen / Victor W.
Henderson.
      p.   cm.
Includes bibliographical references and index.
ISBN 1-85070-078-8 (alk. paper)
1. Brain – Diseases – Hormone therapy.
2. Estrogen – Therapeutic use.   I. Title
    [DNLM: 1. Brain Diseases – therapy.
2. Brain – drug effects.   3. Cognition – drug
effects.   4. Estrogen Replacement Therapy.
5. Estrogens – pharmacology.
WL 348 H497h 1999]
RC483.5.H6H46   1999
616.8′0461 – dc21
DNLM/DLC
for Library of Congress   99-40685
                              CIP

British Library Cataloguing in Publication Data
Henderson, Victor W.
    Hormone therapy and the brain : a clinical
perspective on the role of estrogen
    1. Menopause – Hormone therapy.   2. Brain
    – Effect of drugs on   3. Estrogen –
    Physiological effect
    I. Title
    618.1′75′061

    ISBN 1850700788

Published in the USA by
The Parthenon Publishing Group Inc.
One Blue Hill Plaza
PO Box 1564, Pearl River,
New York 10965, USA

Published in the UK and Europe by
The Parthenon Publishing Group Limited
Casterton Hall, Carnforth,
Lancs, LA6 2LA, UK

Copyright © 2000 The Parthenon Publishing Group

Cover illustration reproduced with kind permission of
T. Okhura and the *Journal of the Japanese Menopause
Society*

Typeset by AMA DataSet Ltd., Preston, Lancs, UK
Printed and bound by T. G. Hostench S.A.,
Spain

Contents

Foreword

The role of estrogen and other so-called sex steroids in central nervous system function has attracted scientific attention for some time. It is only recently, however, that clinicians have begun to consider seriously the potential relevance of estrogen to neurological and psychiatric disease. This exciting prospect has insinuated itself into popular consciousness, and emergent scientific data on estrogen often find quick expression in the lay press and other public forums. Increasingly, well-informed women expect their physicians to be conversant not only with the rationale for commonly accepted clinical practice regarding hormone therapy but also with the merits and caveats of more controversial claims. Questions about Alzheimer's disease are as nearly apt to be asked as those about breast cancer.

In health and disease, estrogen influences various aspects of cerebral activity, including activity in brain regions unconcerned with reproductive functions. The purpose of this monograph is to address the effects of estrogen on neurological function. Basic scientific concepts are briefly presented as a backdrop for the interpretation of human studies. Because our knowledge base remains incomplete, much of the summarized research is best viewed as 'preclinical'. In some instances, clinical implications are apparent, but I have not attempted to offer specific practice guidelines.

The intended audience for this volume includes gynecologists, internists and family practitioners, as well as neurologists, psychiatrists and psychologists. The text also serves as an introductory primer on clinical topics for the basic neuroscientist. The focus is on consequences of estrogen depletion and estrogen replacement after the menopause, with a particular emphasis on cognition and dementia. Research data more appropriate to other portions of the life span are included to illustrate the broader impact of estrogen on neurological function.

The need for a monograph on clinically relevant aspects of hormone therapy and the brain was recognized and brought to my attention by David Bloomer, the prescient Managing Director for Parthenon Publishing and brought to fruition by Dinah Alam, the patient Medical Editor. My own research in the area of estrogen and the brain has focused on clinical and epidemiological aspects of aging and dementia. I particularly thank my colleagues Annlia Paganini-Hill, Galen Buckwalter, Barbara Cherry and Lon Schneider, who were key collaborators on some of my research pertinent to this volume. Scholarly interactions with other University of Southern California colleagues have directly enhanced my academic environment; these include Roberta Brinton, Caleb Finch, Carol McCleary, Carol Miller, Daniel Mishell, Jr, Gail Murdock, Donna Shoupe, Richard Thompson and Leslie Weiner. From time to time, my intellectual milieu has been enriched by debate and discussions with others, including Stanley Birge, Daniel Dorsa, Martin Farlow, Walter Kukull, Rogerio Lobo, Bruce McEwen, Bruce Miller, Frederick Naftolin, Barbara Sherwin, James Simpkins and Leon Speroff. Drs Lobo, Simpkins and Speroff generously commented on the manuscript. Support for my research has come from grants by the National Institutes of Health, the Alzheimer's Association, the French Foundation for Alzheimer Research, and Wyeth–Ayerst Laboratories; from the Bowles Center for Alzheimer's and Related Diseases; and from generous gifts by private donors.

I would like to thank the publishers and authors who have so kindly allowed us to reproduce their figures.

I am especially grateful for the continuous support and continual encouragement of my wife Barbara and the indulgence of my children Gregory, Geoffrey, Stephanie and Nicole. It is my family to whom this book is dedicated.

Victor W. Henderson
Los Angeles

1
Overview

Estrogens are endogenous steroid hormones whose effects extend far beyond well-recognized roles in female reproductive physiology. Menopause, with a concomitant loss of ovarian estrogen production[1] (Figure 1.1), occurs at a median age of 51 years[2], and in the absence of hormone therapy – often loosely referred to as hormone *replacement* therapy – many women will spend about 40% of their adult lives in a state of relative estrogen depletion[3] (Figure 1.2).

Whether estrogen depletion (a physiological description) represents estrogen deficiency (a medical disorder warranting treatment) remains a matter of scientific investigation and public policy debate. There are clear health consequences to hormonal changes associated with the menopause, just as there are with decisions to seek or shun hormone therapy. Physicians' and women's attitudes toward the use of hormone therapy vary from one country to another, and patterns of usage also vary considerably[4]. Usage is most prevalent in the United States, where the most common prescription medication is for postmenopausal estrogen.

With regard to the brain, the absence of ovarian estrogen production after the menopause does not, itself, prove estrogen deficiency. Indeed, estrogen levels within the cerebrospinal fluid appear not to change substantially with age[5], but the extent to which spinal fluid levels reflect central nervous system requirements is unsettled.

Estrogen is by no means the only sex steroid germane to the older woman. Like estrogens, both progestogens and androgens affect brain function. For women with a uterus, estrogen therapy almost always includes a progestational agent to oppose the effect of estrogen on endometrial proliferation. Menopause, particularly surgically induced menopause, may be accompanied by mild reductions in androgen production. Many clinicians in fact advocate androgens in delimited circumstances for their postmenopausal patients[6], for example, as treatment for diminished libido. A gradual decline in androgen production observed in the aging male[7] also has health consequences for men. A reduction in levels of

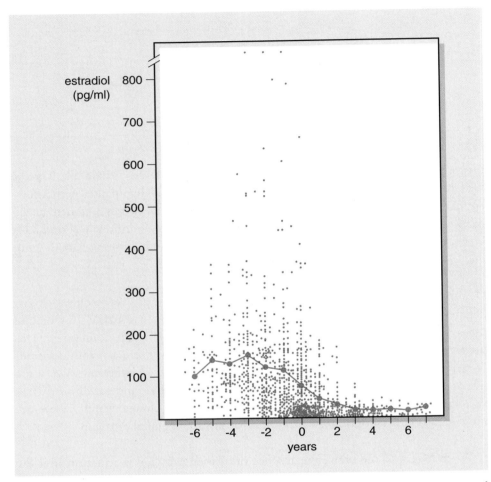

Figure 1.1. Individual and mean plasma levels of estradiol during the perimenopausal and postmenopausal period. Data are from 483 women, ages 45 to 57 years, who had no known endometrial or ovarian pathology and who were not receiving hormone replacement therapy. 0 represents the time of the last menstrual bleeding. The figure indicates that circulating estrogen levels fall dramatically within 4 years of the last menstrual period. Redrawn with permission from reference 1

dehydroepiandrosterone, an androgenic steroid that also serves as an estrogen precursor, has attracted considerable notice in the gerontological literature[8]. Some steroids are synthesized within the central nervous system by glial cells independently of peripheral sources. The term 'neurosteroids' has been applied to these endogenously produced hormones[9], a group that includes pregnenolone, dehydroepiandrosterone and progesterone.

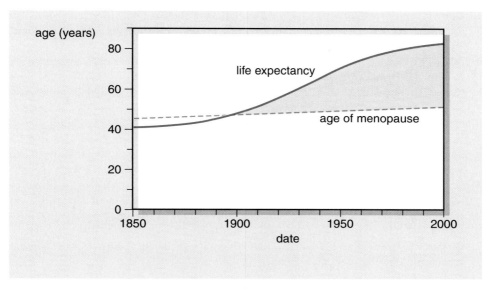

Figure 1.2. Secular trends in female life expectancy during the past 150 years. Prior to the turn of the 20th century, most women did not survive to the age of menopause. Now a woman can expect to live three decades or more after the menopause. Redrawn with permission from reference 3

Despite the theoretical importance of other steroids, this monograph focuses on estrogen to the near exclusion of other hormones. Estrogen depletion in women is more profound than androgen depletion (in women or men), and estrogen therapy is far more prevalent than androgen therapy. Clinical implications of estrogen therapy are therefore more immediate. It is of equal importance that, when compared to estrogen, neurologically relevant data for androgens, progesterone and other gonadal steroids remain fragmentary and rudimentary. This situation is changing, however, and in years ahead any discussion of hormone therapy and the brain will necessarily devote substantial attention to these other important compounds.

REFERENCES

1. Trévoux R, De Brux J, Castanier M, Nahoul K, Soule J-P, Scholler R. Endometrium and plasma hormone profile in the peri-menopause and postmenopause. *Maturitas*, 1986;8: 309–26
2. McKinlay SM, Brambilla DJ, Posner JG. The normal menopause transition. *Maturitas* 1992;14:103–15

3. Cope E. Physical changes associated with the post-menopausal years. In Campbell S, ed. *The Management of the Menopause and Post-Menopausal Years*. Lancaster, UK: MTP Press, 1976

4. Jolleys JV, Olesen F. A comparative study of prescribing of hormone replacement therapy in USA and Europe. *Maturitas* 1996;23:47–53

5. Molnár G, Kassai-Bazsa Z. Gonadotropin, ACTH, prolactin, sexual steroid and cortisol levels in postmenopausal women's cerebrospinal fluid (CSF). *Arch Gerontol Geriatr* 1997;24: 269–80

6. Sands R, Studd J. Exogenous androgens in postmenopausal women. *Am J Med* 1995;98 (Suppl 1A):76S–9S

7. Vermeulen A. Androgens in the aging male. *J Clin Endocrinol Metab* 1991;73:221–4

8. Berr C, Lafont S, Debuire B, Dartigues J-F, Baulieu E-E. Relationships of dehydro-epiandrosterone sulfate in the elderly with functional, psychological, and mental status, and short-term mortality: a French community-based study. *Proc Natl Acad Sci USA* 1996:93: 13410–5

9. Baulieu EE. Neurosteroids: of the nervous system, by the nervous system, for the nervous system. *Rec Progr Hormone Res* 1997;52:1–32

2
Estrogen and the brain

ESTROGEN PRODUCTION AND METABOLISM

Steroid hormones include estrogens, progestogens, androgens and corticoids. Each shares a basic structure of three hexane rings and one pentane ring (Figure 2.1). Estrogens, progestogens and androgens are produced by gonadal tissues and have prominent roles in reproductive functions; collectively they are referred to as sex steroids or gonadal steroids. Estrogens and progestogens are sometimes also known as ovarian steroids or female sex hormones. This designation, however, is slightly misleading: estrogens and progesterone arise in tissues other than the ovaries; the 'male sex hormone' testosterone is also produced by the ovaries, albeit in small quantities; and estrogen has important functions in men as well as women.

Estrogens are derived from cholesterol via precursor androgenic steroids (androstenedione or testosterone) (Figure 2.2). The principal natural estrogens are 17β-estradiol, estrone and estriol; but estrogen metabolites may have restricted biological roles in some cells[1]. During a woman's reproductive years, the most important circulating estrogen is estradiol, produced in the ovaries by granulosa cells of the developing follicle and corpus luteum; small amounts of estradiol also arise in peripheral target tissues through local effects of the enzyme aromatase acting on testosterone. Circulating levels of estradiol vary during the menstrual cycle, with peaks during the follicular phase prior to ovulation and during the luteal phase after ovulation[2,3] (Table 2.1). Progesterone, produced by the corpus luteum, also peaks during the luteal phase. Estrogen and progesterone levels are lowest during the menstrual phase of the cycle (Figure 2.3). Most estrogens circulate tightly bound to a carrier glycoprotein known as sex hormone binding globulin, or loosely bound to serum albumin, and only the free hormone is biologically active.

Ovarian steroidogenesis is under the control of two gonadotropins released from the anterior lobe of the pituitary gland: luteinizing hormone and follicle

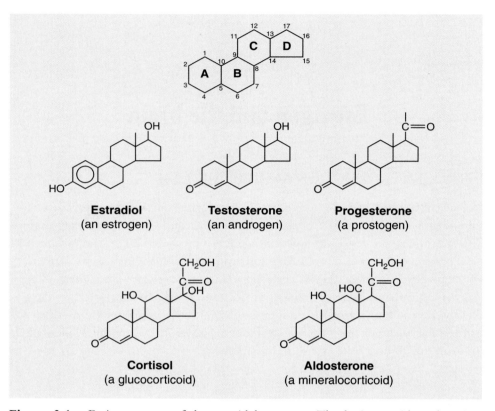

Figure 2.1. Basic structure of the steroid hormones. The basic steroid nucleus is a four-ring cyclopentaneophenanthrene structure. Carbon atoms are numbered as shown, beginning with the A ring. Estrogens have 18 carbon atoms and androgens have 19 carbons; the progestogens, glucocorticoids and mineralocorticoids each contain 21 carbons. Structures of exemplars from each group are shown

Table 2.1. Serum levels of principal estrogens during adult life. Adapted from references 2 and 3

	Approximate normal range (pg/ml)	
Reproductive status	*Estradiol*	*Estrone*
Follicular phase of menstrual cycle	25–600	30–200
Luteal phase of menstrual cycle	100–300	70–100
Pregnancy, third trimester*	10 000–40 000	2000–30 000
Postmenopausal	5–25	30–70

*During pregnancy, levels of estriol in the maternal circulation are intermediate between those of estradiol and estrone

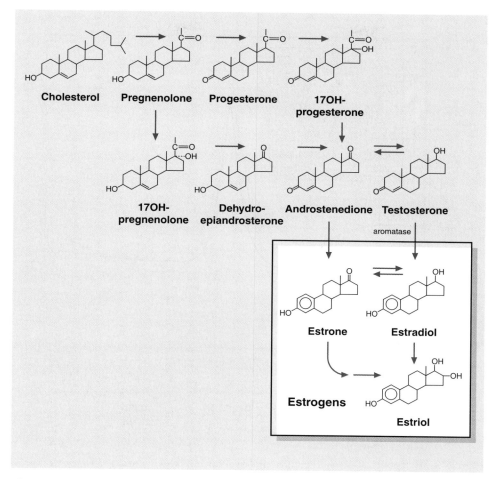

Figure 2.2. Estrogen biosynthesis. Estrogens are formed from cholesterol via androgen precursors in the ovaries and adrenal glands

stimulating hormone (Figure 2.4). These are secreted from pituitary cells called gonadotropes in response to pulsatile stimulation by gonadotropin releasing hormone (GnRH). Cell bodies of GnRH neurons are in the hypothalamus, and GnRH reaches the gonadotropes by way of the pituitary portal circulation. Within the maturing ovarian follicle and the ensuing corpus luteum, androgenic steroids produced by thecal cells are converted to estradiol in granulosa cells that surround the oocyte (Figure 2.3).

After release into the systemic circulation, estradiol is rapidly transformed by the liver to estrone. Estrone is also formed peripherally from androstenedione secreted primarily by the adrenal cortex, with conversion occurring within

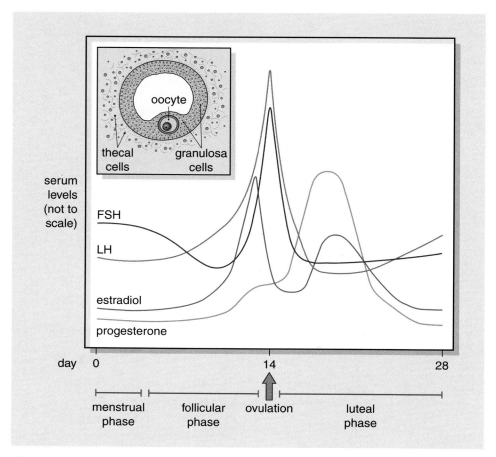

Figure 2.3. Levels of gonadotropins and ovarian hormones during the normal menstrual cycle. Luteinizing hormone (LH) stimulates androgen production in thecal cells of the developing follicle. At the same time, follicle stimulating hormone (FSH) induces estrogen production in the granulosa cells through the aromatization of androgen precursors. Ovulation follows the LH surge at about day 14 of the menstrual cycle. During the luteal phase, both progesterone and estrogen are produced by the granulosa cells. In the absence of fertilization, declines in estrogen and progesterone production lead to menstruation. Insert: Schematic view of an ovarian follicle at the late follicular stage of development, showing thecal and granulosa layers. After ovulation, the oocyte and surrounding granulosa cells become the corpus luteum

adipose tissue and other extraglandular sources. Both estradiol and estrone can be converted to estriol, a less active estrogen present in high concentrations in the urine. Other estrogen metabolites are excreted in the urine and bile as water-soluble sulfate and glucuronide conjugates.

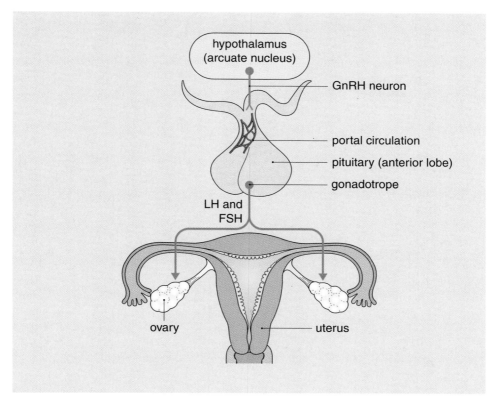

Figure 2.4. Hypothalamic regulation of ovarian estrogen production. Neurons projecting from the arcuate nucleus of the hypothalamus release gonadotropin releasing hormone (GnRH) into the portal circulation of the anterior pituitary gland. In response, luetinizing hormone (LH) and follicle stimulating hormone (FSH) are secreted from pituitary gonadotropes to regulate sex steroid production within the ovary and the menstrual cycle

Enormous quantities of estradiol, estriol and estrone are produced during pregnancy (Table 2.1); estrogen production by the placenta involves precursors derived from both the mother and the fetus. After the menopause, virtually all estrogens arise by the peripheral conversion of androgenic precursors[4].

THE BRAIN AS AN ESTROGEN TARGET ORGAN

Reproductive tissues (uterus, vagina, Fallopian tubes, breast) are key estrogen targets, but estrogen also has clear-cut effects on bone, vascular endothelium, skin and other tissues (Figure 2.5). Of these non-reproductive sites, none is more important than the nervous system. Unique among body organs, the brain is

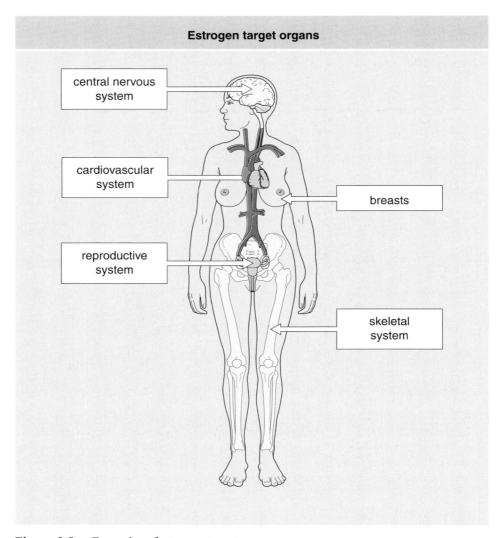

Figure 2.5. Examples of estrogen target organs

focally organized to an extraordinary degree. Individual neurons differ in form, biochemical composition and physiological properties. All neurons are massively interconnected with other neurons, and many maintain connections with sensory organs or muscle fibers. Activation of discrete populations of neurons leads to widely divergent effects depending on which neurons have been activated and on the activity profile of interconnected neurons. It has long been recognized that estrogen affects the hypothalamus and anterior pituitary to modulate control of ovarian function and the menstrual cycle. However, the importance of estrogen on different aspects of brain activity far exceeds its regulatory role in reproductive

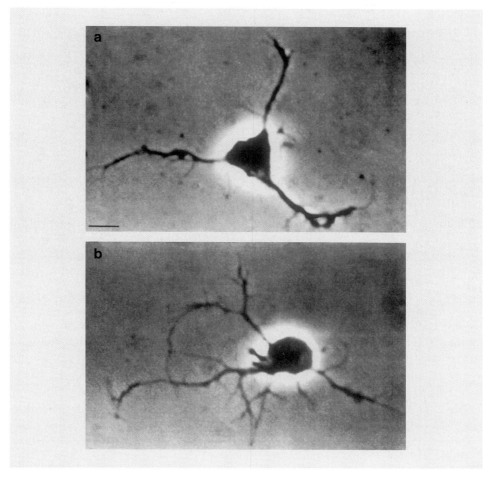

Figure 2.6. Estrogen and the growth of neuronal processes in primary culture. Dissociated neurons obtained from the cortex of fetal rats were grown in culture for one day in the absence (**a**) or presence (**b**) of estrogen. Reproduced with permission from reference 10

physiology. Indeed, throughout the life span, ovarian steroids play crucial roles in the formation, maintenance and remodelling of neuronal circuits in the brain[5–10] (Figures 2.6, 2.7 and 2.8).

Generally speaking, not only does estrogen act as a classic hormone on distant target tissues (endocrine activity), but estrogen can also bind to receptors on cells of origin (autocrine activity) or diffuse locally to influence contiguous cells (paracrine activity). With respect to the nervous system, estrogen is not synthesized by neurons. Astrocytes, however, can produce estradiol *in vitro*[11], and

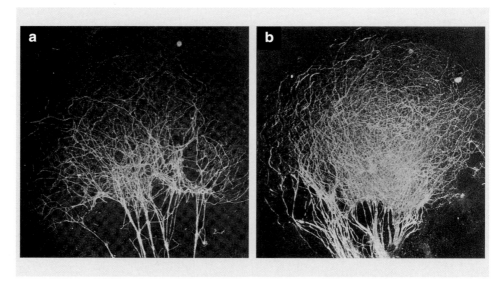

Figure 2.7. Estrogen and the growth of neuronal processes in brain explants. Explants of developing brain (preoptic area of the newborn mouse) cultured in serum not supplemented with estradiol show less exuberant outgrowth of nerve processes (**a**) than do explants cultured in serum with supplemental estradiol (**b**). Reproduced with permission from reference 5

Table 2.2. Organizational effects of early hormone exposure on brain structures: examples of sex-associated morphological differences. From reference 16

Number of neurons
Size of individual neurons
Number of neuronal and synaptic organelles
Pattern of dendritic branching
Number of dendritic spines on a dendritic branch
Number, type and distribution of synapses
Density of axonal innervation
Regional volume of neuronal groups

paracrine effects – in addition to endocrine effects – are therefore possible in the brain. In addition, neurons[12] and astrocytes[11] that contain the enzyme aromatase can convert circulating testosterone to estradiol *in situ*. This process is especially important developmentally, but the same mechanism is presumably germane to mature organisms[13].

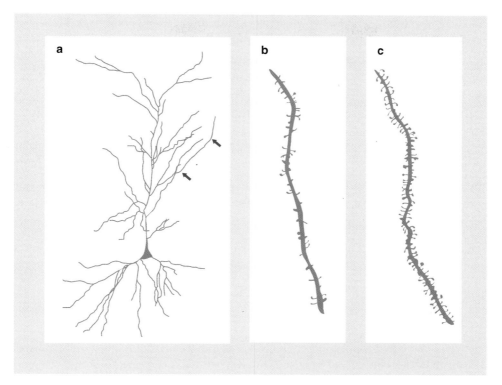

Figure 2.8. Hormone replacement and dendritic spine density in the CA1 region of the hippocampus. (**a**) Representative pyramidal neuron showing examples of apical dendrites (arrowheads). (**b** and **c**) Camera lucida drawings of apical dendrites taken from adult female rats which had undergone ovariectomy; (b) is from an animal that did not receive hormone replacement and (c) is from an animal that received estradiol plus progesterone. Dendritic spines, believed to represents points of excitatory synaptic contact along the apical dendrites, are more numerous in (c). Reproduced with permission from reference 9

Within the brain, sex steroid actions can be conceptualized as irreversible (organizational effects) or transient (activational effects)[14], although the validity of this dichotomous characterization has been challenged[15]. Organizational effects are known to occur prenatally and in the immediate postnatal period. Other permanent effects may also take place during puberty. Organizational effects presumably represent 'hard-wired' patterns of neuronal connections[16] (Table 2.2). Short-lived activational effects can occur at any age.

In studies of adult laboratory rats, sex-specific behavioral differences are largely determined by perinatal exposures to sex hormones. These differences include exploratory and socially aggressive behaviors, as well as specific reproductive behaviors. Other behaviors, such as learning performance that depends on spatial cues, are also influenced by the prenatal steroid environment[17]. In the absence of early exposure to gonadal steroids, the animal will develop the pattern of neuronal organization and the behaviors typical of female adults. For mammals, the female pattern of development is thus the default pattern. Interestingly, fetal masculinization occurs through actions of estrogen produced locally from androgen precursors. In the developing male, testosterone released by the fetal testes circulates to the brain. There, testosterone is aromatized to estradiol, and patterns of neuronal growth and differentiation are permanently altered (an organizational effect of androgens acting through estrogen). Despite high levels in the maternal circulation, maternal estrogens are tightly bound to α-fetoprotein and do not reach the fetus. Sexual differentiation of the human nervous system is likely to occur in a similar manner. As an example, early exposure to androgens appears to influence gender-associated toy preferences later in childhood[18].

MECHANISMS OF ESTROGEN ACTION WITHIN THE BRAIN

Receptor-mediated effects

Estrogens are small lipophilic molecules, which in their unbound state diffuse readily into the central nervous system. Estrogen has the potential to influence brain function in widespread and discrete fashions (Table 2.3). As is the case for other steroid hormones, many key estrogen effects are receptor-mediated and occur at the level of the genome, where estrogen regulates gene expression to

Table 2.3. Estrogen effects on the brain: possible mechanisms of action

Mediators of direct effects on neurons
Intranuclear receptors
Membrane receptors
Intracellular processes not requiring receptor binding

Mediators of indirect effects on neurons
Direct effects on other interconnecting neurons
Effects on glial cells
Effects on the immune system
Effects on cerebral blood flow
    short-term effects on vascular reactivity and the vascular endothelium
    short-term effects on coagulation
    effects on lipids and atheromatous build-up
Effects on cerebral metabolism

Table 2.4. Tissue-specific and cell-specific effects of estrogens: possible mechanisms for selective actions

---

Specific genomic effects (transcriptional regulation of target genes)
Different estrogens and estrogen metabolites
Different distributions of estrogen receptors (ERα, ERβ) and receptor subtypes
Different adaptor proteins, which interact with the estrogen–receptor complex
Different DNA response elements within regulatory regions of the target gene
Different transcription factors that bind to regulatory regions of the target gene

Specific non-genomic effects
Different estrogens and estrogen metabolites
Different distributions of putative membrane receptors
Different effects on pathways and processes requiring neither membrane nor nuclear receptors

---

affect the transcription of specific proteins[19]. A high degree of regulatory complexity modulates the process by which the ligand–receptor complex ultimately impacts transcription, implying that there are numerous ways in which cell-specific estrogen effects are realized (Table 2.4).

After entering the cell, an estrogen molecule passes to the nucleus, where it binds to a high-affinity receptor protein. The estrogen receptor has hormone-binding, DNA-binding and regulatory domains. Hormone binding initiates a series of events involving complexed proteins that structurally transform and activate the receptor. Two identical ligand–receptor complexes then join (dimerize) and together bind to a specific DNA sequence – the estrogen response element – in the regulatory region of a target gene. This interaction regulates transcription of a downstream genomic sequence; the resultant messenger RNA is eventually translated as a specific protein product (Figure 2.9).

Within the hormone-binding domain of the estrogen receptor, two regions can exert control over gene transcription. These are referred to as transcriptional activation function (TAF-1 and TAF-2) regions. Adaptor proteins known as co-activators and co-repressors can interact with these transcriptional activation function regions, and different adaptor proteins are found in different cells. As further described below, different tissues and individual cells may also vary according to the type of estrogen receptor and the availability of transcription factors that bind to DNA. Other regulatory control involves the particular DNA response sites to which the estrogen–receptor complex binds.

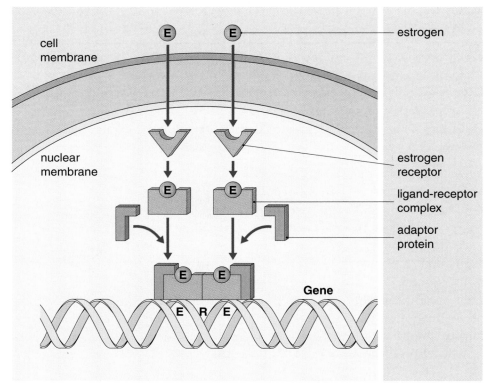

Figure 2.9. Transcriptional regulation by estrogen. In this conceptual scheme, binding of estrogen (E) to its receptor occurs in the cell nucleus. Binding leads to a dissociation of complexed proteins and a conformational change in the receptor shape. Two ligand–receptor complexes join to form a dimer, which in association with adaptor proteins attaches to the estrogen response element (ERE) site on the genome, resulting in transcriptional regulation of a downstream gene

Receptor types

Two classes of intracellular estrogen receptors have been identified, termed alpha and beta, or ERα and ERβ[20–22]. The DNA-binding domains of the two receptor types are highly homologous and the ligand-binding domains somewhat less so[20]. Different estrogens have different binding affinities for ERα and ERβ[23]. For many estrogenic molecules, binding is similar for the two receptors, but there are notable exceptions (Table 2.5). The distribution of receptor types – as inferred from the regional expression of receptor messenger RNA – differs in different tissues[23], and this variability is certain to contribute to selective actions of estrogens in different target areas. Estrogen receptors also exist in different iso-forms[24,25] (minor variations in protein sequence), and, interestingly, isoforms of ERβ are known to be distributed differently in different target tissues[25].

16

Table 2.5. Relative binding affinities of select compounds at the alpha (ERα) and beta estrogen receptor (ERβ). The reference compound is 17β-estradiol, where the relative binding affinity is defined as 100. Data from reference 23

Compound	Relative binding affinity	
	ERα	ERβ
Estradiol	100	100
Diethylstilbestrol*	468	295
Coumestrol*	94	185
Estrone	60	37
Zearalanol*	16	14
Estriol	14	21
Tamoxifen[†]	7	6
Genistein*	5	36
Dehydroepiandrosterone	0.04	0.07
Bisphenol A*	0.05	0.33
Methoxychlor*	0.01	0.13
Testosterone	< 0.01	< 0.01
Progesterone	< 0.001	< 0.001

*Dietary estrogens, including synthetic estrogens, phytoestrogens and mycoestrogens; [†]a selective estrogen receptor modulator

Some neurons express ERα, some express ERβ and some express neither receptor; in other regions both receptor types co-exist[23,26]. Within the hippocampus and cerebral cortex, for example, the predominant receptor type is ERβ[27] (Figure 2.10). Theoretically, estrogen activation within a neuron that expresses both ERα and ERβ could lead to both homodimer (ERα/ERα and ERβ/ERβ) and heterodimer (ERα/ERβ) formation, thus increasing the potential for selective activation at DNA response elements. The brain also possesses receptors for androgens, and there is a partial overlap between neuronal subsets that contain androgen and estrogen receptors[28].

Selective estrogen receptor modulators and transcriptional control

Some compounds have antiestrogenic effects in some tissues and estrogen-like effects in others (Figure 2.11). For example, both tamoxifen and raloxifene act as an estrogen antagonist in the breast but have partial agonist activity on blood lipids and bone density. Tamoxifen, but not raloxifene, exerts estrogenic effects on the endometrium of the uterus[29,30]. Other combinations of tissue selectivity are

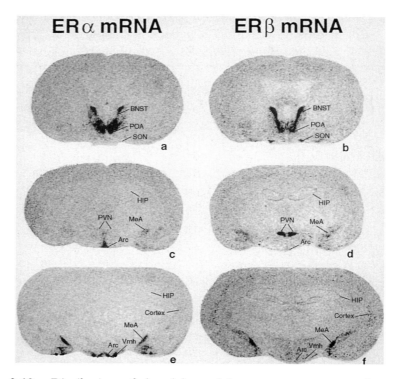

Figure 2.10. Distribution of the alpha and beta estrogen receptors in rat brain. Autoradiograms of cells in the rat brain that contain messenger RNA (mRNA) for the alpha receptor (**a**, **c** and **e**) and beta receptor (**b**, **d** and **f**). Coronal sections a vs. b, c vs. d, and e vs. f are adjacent. Arc, arcuate nucleus; BNST, bed nucleus of the stria terminalis; Cortex, cerebral cortex; HIP, hippocampus; MeA, medial amygdala; POA, preoptic area; PVN, paraventricular nucleus; SON, supraoptic nucleus; Vmh, ventromedial hypothalamic nucleus. Reproduced with permission from reference 27

possible, and one experimental compound (Imperial Chemical Industries 164384) is a pure antiestrogen, blocking receptor-mediated effects of estradiol in all tissues studied. The term selective estrogen receptor modulator (SERM) has been applied to tissue-specific agents.

Like other estrogenic compounds, a SERM binds to the hormone-binding domain of the estrogen receptor, and each SERM appears to induce a unique conformational change in the receptor[31,32]. Available evidence indicates that SERMs do not block binding of the ligand–receptor complex to DNA[31,33]. DNA binding can occur not only at the estrogen response element in the promotor region of the gene but also at other DNA sites[1,34]. Adaptor proteins can be crucial to this interaction[1], and different tissues have different adaptors.

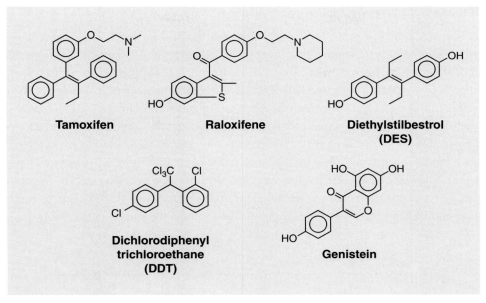

Figure 2.11. Examples of non-steroidal compounds having estrogenic or antiestrogenic activity. Shown are structures of two selective estrogen receptor modulators (SERMs) tamoxifen and raloxifene, the synthetic estrogen diethylstilbestrol (DES), the pesticide dichlorodiphenyl trichloroethane (DDT) and the phytoestrogen genistein

Selective receptor modulation also involves the transcriptional activation function regions of the estrogen receptor. For example, a side-chain of the raloxifene molecule blocks TAF-2, which is located within the hormone-binding domain of the receptor and is required for gene transcription in the breast or endometrium[32]. In contrast, raloxifene does not interfere with TAF-1, located in the regulatory domain and required for gene transcription in bone.

It is important to recognize that the binding of a ligand to the estrogen receptor can activate or inhibit gene transcription depending on the estrogen or SERM in question, depending on whether binding is with the alpha or beta receptor and depending on whether the ligand–receptor complex in turn binds at the estrogen response element or a different DNA region[34]. Although ligand–receptor interactions usually involve direct binding with the genome (for example, at the estrogen response element), transcriptional control is sometimes mediated through transcriptional factors, which are themselves attached to a particular DNA response element[34,35]. For example, estrogen may influence a signal transduction pathway involving cyclic AMP by increasing the phosphorylation of a transcription factor required for neuronal gene expression[35,36].

Effects not mediated by intranuclear receptors

As discussed in the preceding paragraphs, the distribution within different brain areas of intranuclear estrogen receptors provides an imprecise guide to the regional specificity of estrogen actions. To add to this complexity, some estrogen effects appear too rapidly to be mediated by genomic activation and are presumed to require binding to specific protein receptors on the cell membrane[37] (Table 2.4 and Figure 2.12). Such actions include changes in neuronal excitability and the stimulation of neurotransmitter release. Membrane receptors have yet to be characterized biochemically and may or may not differ from intranuclear receptors. They are thought to be linked to ion channels and neurotransmitter receptors both directly and through second messenger systems[37]. In the hippocampus, a brain region critical to learning and memory, only a subset of neurons in the adult brain

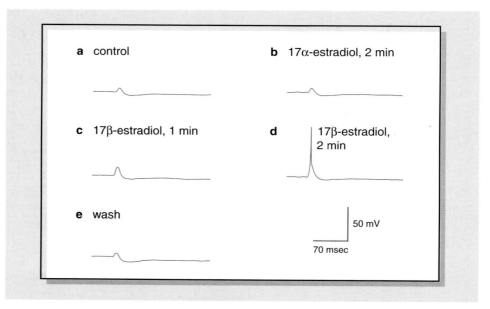

Figure 2.12. Rapid effects of estrogen on the excitatory post–synaptic potential (EPSP) of a pyramidal neuron in the CA1 region of the hippocampus of an adult female rat. (**a**) In this hippocampal slice preparation, an intracellular recording electrode detected a small EPSP (positive deflection) when synaptic input to the neuron was activated. (**b**) Adding 17α-estradiol to the artificial cerebrospinal fluid bathing the hippocampal slice had no effect on EPSP amplitude after 2 mins. (**c**) In contrast to the negative effect of 17α-estradiol, 17β-estradiol added to the bath at a concentration of 10^{-8} M increased EPSP amplitude in response to synaptic activation after 1 min. (**d**) Two mins after 17β-estradiol was added, the threshold for an action potential (large, sharp positive deflection) was reached. (**e**) Washing out the 17β-estradiol reduced the amplitude of the evoked EPSP to that seen under control conditions. Reproduced with permission from reference 55

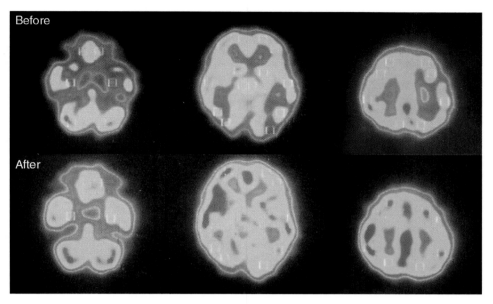

Figure 2.13. Estrogen effect on regional blood flow in the brain. Regional blood flow before (top row) and after (bottom row) beginning estrogen therapy (1.25 mg per day conjugated estrogens) in a woman with premature menopause. Quantitative blood flow measurements were obtained using single photon emission computed tomography. Horizontal (axial) slices are shown for three levels of the brain, where regional blood flow is depicted on a red–orange–yellow–green–blue false color scale (greater to lesser). Greater flow is seen in many brain regions during estrogen therapy (bottom row). Reproduced with permission from reference 51

appear to possess intracellular estrogen receptors[26,38]. However, estrogen prominently affects the morphology and physiological properties of specific populations of hippocampal neurons[39–45] (Figures 2.8 and 2.12). Changes in hippocampal neurons induced by estrogen are sex specific and are modified by early developmental exposures[46].

Other estrogen influences on brain function occur indirectly (Table 2.3). Receptor-mediated effects in one neuronal population can influence the function of neurons in a distant brain region with which it maintains axodendritic contact. Estrogen actions on astroglial cells also influence neuronal function. Glia, like neurons, can express estrogen receptors, and estrogen promotes the extension of astrocytic processes[47,48]. Other indirect effects can occur through the modulation of immunocompetent cells[49], the enhancement of cerebral blood flow[50,51] (Figure 2.13), or the augmentation of glucose utilization by the brain[52].

DIETARY ESTROGENS

A large number of compounds display estrogen-like physiological properties[53]. Strictly speaking, natural and synthetic substances that lack the basic steroid structure are not true estrogens, but they are commonly referred to as such. A basic requirement of all these compounds appears to be the presence or functional equivalent of the aromatic 'A' ring of the basic steroid structure (Figures 2.1 and 2.11). Effects of dietary estrogens can be receptor- or non-receptor-mediated. At the receptor level, a dietary estrogen can show differential binding affinities for the two estrogen receptor types (ERα and ERβ)[23] (Table 2.5). Dietary estrogens can evince antiestrogenic as well as estrogenic effects. For humans and for wildlife, dietary estrogens can have deleterious health-related consequences, but there may also be beneficial effects[54–56]. Behavioral effects[57,58] of dietary estrogens are linked to the ability of these compounds to bind to estrogen receptors in the brain[57].

Estrogen exposure through oral ingestion is to some extent unavoidable (Table 2.6). Endogenous estrogens are found in meat products, as are synthetic compounds such as diethylstilbestrol (DES) used to enhance livestock growth. Pesticides (e.g. dichlorodiphenyl trichloroethane (DDT) and methoxychlor) and other industrial compounds (e.g. bisphenol A) are other dietary estrogens. Phthalates, used in the manufacture of plastics, are ubiquitous in the environment[59]. Fungi can produce estrogens (mycoestrogens), and livestock that ingest zearalanol, a mycoestrogen found in moldy grain, can develop infertility.

The best recognized dietary estrogens are the phytoestrogens, or plant estrogens, contained in many grains, fruits and vegetables. These include isoflavones,

Table 2.6. Dietary estrogens

Natural, endogenous estrogens (meat products)
Synthetic estrogens (e.g. diethylstilbestrol (DES), administered to livestock)
Industrial compounds
    pesticides (e.g. dichlorodiphenyl trichloroethane (DDT) and methoxychlor)
    chemicals used in the manufacture of plastics (e.g. bisphenol A)
Mycoestrogens (fungal metabolites, e.g. zearalanol in mold-infected grains)
Natural plant estrogens (phytoestrogens)
    isoflavones (e.g. in soybeans)
    flavones (in many fruits and vegetables)
    coumestans (e.g. in bean sprouts)
    lignans (e.g. in linseed oil)

---

flavones, coumestans and lignans. Isoflavones are found in high concentrations in legumes and grains. Tofu and other soy products are a rich source of the isoflavones genistein and daidzein. Flavones are ubiquitous in many fruits and vegetables. Coumestan, a coumestrol, is found in bean sprouts, and lignans are found in linseed oil and in other cereals and vegetables.

Some dietary estrogens (e.g. DES; Table 2.5) are highly potent. Most, however, are not. Nevertheless, even a relatively low-potency estrogen is highly relevant when naturally present in high quantities (e.g. isoflavones in soy beans) or when concentrated at higher levels of the food chain (e.g. lipophilic compounds such as DDT).

There is epidemiological evidence that phytoestrogen consumption ameliorates menopausal symptoms and reduces the risk of cardiovascular disease and certain other age-associated illnesses[60]. For example, menopausal symptoms are relatively mild in many Asian countries, an observation that may be explained by evidence that dietary soy can reduce hot flushes[61]. For some reported associations, however, clinical trial data are sparse or lacking. Moreover, as briefly discussed in Chapters 4 and 5, it is possible that some phytoestrogens are actually detrimental to neurological function[58,62,63]

REFERENCES

1. Yang NN, Venugopalan M, Hardikar S, Glasebrook A. Identification of an estrogen response element activated by metabolites of 17β-estadiol and raloxifene. *Science* 1996;273: 1222–5
2. Soules MR, Bremner WJ. The menopause and climacteric: endocrinologic basis and associated symptomatology. *J Am Geriatr Soc* 1982;30:547–61
3. Speroff L, Glass RH, Kase NG. *Clinical Gynecologic Endocrinology and Infertility*, 5th edn. Baltimore: Williams & Wilkins, 1994
4. Judd HL, Judd GE, Lucas WE, Yen SSC. Endocrine function of the postmenopausal ovary: concentration of androgens and estrogens in ovarian and peripheral vein blood. *J Clin Endocrinol Metab* 1974;39:1020–4
5. Toran-Allerand CD, Gerlach JL, McEwen BS. Audiographic localization of [³H]estradiol related to steroid responsiveness in cultures of the newborn mouse hypothalamus and pre-optic area. *Brain Res* 1980;184:517–22
6. Matsumoto A. Synaptogenic action of sex steroids in developing and adult neuroendocrine brain. *Psychoneuroendocrinology* 1991;16:25–40
7. Chung SK, Pfaff DW, Cohen RS. Estrogen-induced alterations in synaptic morphology in the midbrain central gray. *Exp Brain Res* 1988;69:522–30
8. Toran-Allerand CD. Organotypic culture of the developing cerebral cortex and hypothalamus: relevance to sexual differentiation. *Psychoneuroendocrinology* 1991;16:7–24

9. Gould E, Woolley CS, Frankfurt M, McEwen BS. Gonadal steroids regulate dendritic spine density in hippocampal pyramidal cells in adulthood. *J Neurosci* 1990;10:1286–91

10. Brinton RD, Proffitt P, Tran J, Luu R. Equilin, a principal component of the estrogen replacement therapy Premarin, increases the growth of cortical neurons via an NMDA receptor-dependent mechanism. *Exp Neurol* 1997;147:211–20

11. Zwain IH, Yen SSC, Cheng CY. Astrocytes cultured *in vitro* produce estradiol-17β and express aromatase cytochrome P-450 (P-450 AROM) mRNA. *Biochim Biophys Acta* 1997;1334:338–48

12. Naftolin F, Horvath TL, Jakab RL, Leranth C, Harada N, Balhazart J. Aromatase immuno-reactivity in axon terminals of the vertebrate brain. *Neuroendocrinology* 1996;63: 149–55

13. Michael RP, Bonsall RW, Rees HD. The nuclear accumulation of [³H]testosterone and [³H]estradiol in the brain of the female primate: evidence for the aromatization hypothesis. *Endocrinology* 1986;118:1935–44

14. Young WC, Goy RW, Phoenix CH. Hormones and sexual behavior. *Science* 1964;143: 212–8

15. Arnold AP, Breedlove SM. Organizational and activational effects of sex steroids on brain and behavior: a reanalysis. *Horm Behav* 1985;19:469–98

16. MacLusky NJ, Bowlby DA, Brown TJ, Peterson RE, Hochberg RB. Sex and the developing brain: suppression of neuronal estrogen sensitivity by developmental androgen exposure. *Neurochem Res* 1997;22:1395–414

17. Isgor C, Sengelaub DR. Prenatal gonadal steroids affect adult spatial behavior, CA1 and CA3 pyramidal cell morphology in rats. *Horm Behav* 1998;34:183–98

18. Berenbaum SA, Hines M. Early androgens are related to childhood sex-type type preferences. *Psychol Sci* 1992;3:203–6

19. Evans RM. The steroid and thyroid hormone receptor superfamily. *Science* 1988;249: 889–95

20. Kuiper GGJM, Enmark E, Pelto-Huikko M, Nilsson S, Gustafsson J-A. Cloning of a novel estrogen receptor expressed in rat prostate and ovary. *Proc Natl Acad Sci USA* 1996;93: 5925–30

21. Mosselman S, Polman J, Dijkema R. ERβ: identification and characterization of a novel human estrogen receptor. *FEBS Lett* 1996;392:49–53

22. Shughrue PJ, Komm B, Merchenthaler I. The distribution of estrogen receptor-β mRNA in the rat hypothalamus. *Steroids* 1996;61:678–81

23. Kuiper GGJM, Carlsson B, Grandien K, *et al.* Comparison of the ligand binding specificity and transcript tissue distribution of estrogen receptors α and β. *Endocrinology* 1997;138: 863–70

24. Friend KE, Ang LW, Shupnik MA. Estrogen regulates the expression of several different estrogen receptor mRNA isoforms in rat pituitary. *Proc Natl Acad Sci USA* 1995;92: 4367–71

25. Petersen DN, Tkalcevic GT, Koza-Taylor PH, Turi TG, Brown TA. Identification of estrogen receptor β_2, a functional variant of estrogen receptor β expressed in normal rat tissues. *Endocrinology* 1998;139:1082–92

26. Shughrue PJ, Lane MV, Merchenthaler I. Comparative distribution of estrogen receptor-α and -β mRNA in the rat central nervous system. *J Comp Neurol* 1997;388:507–25

27. Shughrue PJ. Estrogen action in the estrogen receptor α-knockout mouse: is this due to ER-β? *Mol Psychiatry* 1998;3:299–302

28. Wood RI, Newman SW. Androgen and estrogen receptors coexist within individual neurons in the brain of the Syrian hamster. *Neuroendocrinology* 1995;62:487–97

29. Sato M, Rippy MK, Bryant HU. Raloxifene, tamoxifen, nafoxidine, or estrogen effects on reproductive and nonreproductive tissues in ovariectomized rats. *FASEB J* 1996;10:905–12

30. Delmas PD, Bjarnason NH, Mitlak BH, *et al.* Effects of raloxifene on bone mineral density, serum cholesterol concentrations, and uterine endometrium in postmenopausal women. *N Engl J Med* 1997;337:1641–7

31. McDonnell DP, Clemm DL, Hermann T, Goldman ME, Pike JW. Analysis of estrogen receptor function *in vitro* reveals three distinct classes of antiestrogens. *Mol Endocrinol* 1995;9:659–69

32. Brzozowski AM, Pike ACW, Dauter Z, *et al.* Molecular basis of agonism and antagonism in the oestrogen receptor. *Nature (London)* 1997;389:753–8

33. Katzenellenbogen JA, O'Malley BW, Katzenellenbogen BS. Tripartite steroid hormone receptor pharmacology: interaction with multiple effector sites as a basis for the cell- and promotor-specific action of these hormones. *Mol Endocrinol* 1996;10:119–31

34. Paech K, Webb P, Kuiper GGJM, *et al.* Differential ligand activation of estrogen receptors ERα and ERβ at AP1 sites. *Science* 1997;277:1508–10

35. Watters JJ, Dorsa DM. Transcriptional effects of estrogen on neuronal neurotensin gene expression involve cAMP/protein kinase A-dependent signaling mechanisms. *J Neurosci* 1998;18:6672–80

36. Panickar KS, Guan G, King MA, Rajakumar G, Simpkins JW. 17β-estradiol attenuates CREB decline in the rat hippocampus following seizure. *J Neurobiol* 1997;33:961–7

37. Wong M, Thompson TL, Moss RL. Nongenomic actions of estrogen in the brain: physiological significance and cellular mechanisms. *Crit Rev Neurobiol* 1996;10:189–203

38. Loy R, Gerlach JL, McEwen BS. Autoradiographic localization of estradiol-binding neurons in the rat hippocampal formation and entorhinal cortex. *Dev Brain Res* 1988;39:245–51

39. Woolley CS, McEwen BS. Roles of estradiol and progesterone in regulation of hippocampal dendritic spine density during the estrous cycle in the rat. *J Comp Neurol* 1993;336:293–306

40. Woolley CS, Weiland NG, McEwen BS, Schwartzkroin PA. Estradiol increases the sensitivity of hippocampal CA1 pyramidal cells to NMDA receptor-mediated synaptic input: correlation with dendritic spine density. *J Neurosci* 1997;17:1848–59

41. Warren SG, Humphreys AG, Juraska JM, Greenough WT. LTP varies across the estrous cycle: enhanced synaptic plasticity in proestrus rats. *Brain Res* 1995;703:26–30

42. Gibbs RB, Hashash A, Johnson DA. Effects of estrogen on potassium-stimulated acetylcholine release in the hippocampus and overlying cortex of adult rats. *Brain Res* 1996;749:143–6

43. Weiland NG. Estradiol selectively regulates agonist binding sites on the N-methyl-D-aspartate receptor complex in the CA1 region of the hippocampus. *Endocrinology* 1992;131:662–8

44. Foy MR, Xu J, Xie X, Brinton RD, Thompson RF, Burger TW. 17β-estradiol enhances NMDA receptor-mediated EPSPs and long-term potentiation. *J Neurophysiol* 1999;81:925–9

45. Wong M, Moss RL. Long-term and short-term electrophysiological effects of estrogen on the synaptic properties of hippocampal CA1 neurons. *J Neurosci* 1992;12:3217–25

46. Lewis C, McEwen BS, Frankfurt M. Estrogen-induction of dendritic spines in ventro-medial hypothalamus and hippocampus: effects of neonatal aromatase blockade and adult GDX. *Dev Brain Res* 1995;87:91–5

47. Santagati S, Melcangi RC, Celotti F, Martini L, Maggi A. Estrogen receptor is expressed in different types of glial cells in culture. *J Neurochem* 1994;63:2058–64

48. Garcia-Segura LM, Chowen JA, Dueñas M, Parducz A, Naftolin F. Gonadal steroids and astroglial plasticity. *Cell Mol Neurobiol* 1997;16:225–37

49. Grossman CJ. Interactions between the gonadal steroids and the immune sytstem. *Science* 1985;227:257–61

50. Belfort MA, Saade GR, Snabes M, *et al*. Hormonal status affects the reactivity of the cerebral vasculature. *Am J Obstet Gynecol* 1995;172:1273–8

51. Ohkura T, Matsuda H, Iwasaki N, *et al*. Effect of estrogen on regional cerebral blood flow in postmenopausal women. *J Jpn Menopause Soc* 1996;4:254–61

52. Bishop J, Simpkins JW. Role of estrogens in peripheral and cerebral glucose utilization. *Rev Neurosci* 1992;3:121–37

53. Katzenellenbogen JA. The structural pervasiveness of estrogenic activity. *Environ Health Perspect* 1995;103(Suppl 7):99–101

54. Colborn T, vom Saal FS, Soto AM. Developmental effects of endocrine-disrupting chemicals in wildlife and humans. *Environ Health Perspect* 1993;101:378–84

55. Davis DL, Bradlow HL, Wolff M, Woodruff T, Hoel DG, Anton-Culver H. Medical hypothesis: xenoestrogens as preventable causes of breast cancer. *Environ Health Perspect* 1993;101:372–7

56. Adlercreutz H. Phytoestrogens: epidemiology and a possible role in cancer protection. *Environ Health Perspect* 1995;103(Suppl 7):103–12

57. vom Saal FS, Nagel SC, Palanza P, Boechler M, Parmigiani S, Welshons WV. Estrogenic pesticides: binding relative to estradiol in MCF-7 cells and effects of exposure during fetal life on subsequent territorial behaviour in male mice. *Toxicol Lett* 1995;77:343–50

58. Whitten PL, Lewis C, Russell E, Naftolin F. Potential adverse effects of phytoestrogens. *J Nutr* 1995;125:771S–6S

59. Jobling S, Reynolds T, White R, Parker MG, Sumpter JP. A variety of environmentally persistent chemicals, including some phthalate plasticizers, are weakly estrogenic. *Environ Health Perspect* 1995;103:582–7

60. Knight DC, Eden JA. Phytoestrogens: a short review. *Maturitas* 1995;22:167–75

61. Albertazzi P, Pansini F, Bonaccorsi G, Zanotti L, Forini E, De Aloysio D. The effect of dietary soy supplementation on hot flushes. *Obstet Gynecol* 1998;91:6–11

62. Rice MM, Graves AB, Larson EB. Estrogen replacement therapy and cognition: role of phytoestrogens [abstr]. *Gerontologist* 1995;35(Suppl 1):169

63. White L, Petrovitch H, Ross GW, Masaki K. Association of mid-life consumption of tofu with late life cognitive impairment and dementia: the Honolulu–Asia Study [abstr]. *Neurobiol Aging* 1996;17(Suppl):S121

64.

3
Mood

Estrogen influences a myriad of brain functions that potentially impact mood and behavior. In general, estrogen appears to have a positive effect on mental outlook[1]. Estrogen administration increases psychological well-being in adolescents with Turner syndrome[2], a sex chromosome anomaly in which phenotypic females with a partial or complete absence of the second X chromosome (45,XO karyotype) fail to undergo spontaneous pubertal maturation. A woman's sense of well-being is heightened during the late follicular stage of the menstrual cycle[3], a time when estradiol levels are elevated but progesterone levels are still low. During the climacteric, estrogen replacement is reported to diminish anxiety and to enhance both mood and mental well-being[4-9].

Rates of bipolar affective disorder are similar for men and women, but women are twice as likely as men to experience depressed mood or suffer major depression[10] (Figure 3.1). The difference in rates of unipolar affective disturbances may

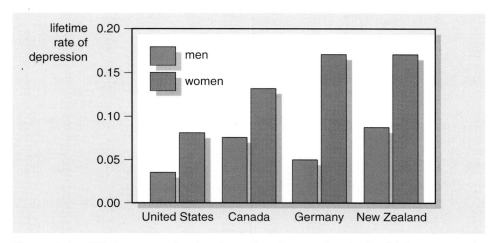

Figure 3.1. Lifetime rate of major depression, by sex. Standardized lifetime rates for men and women ages 26–64 years from the United States (five communities), Edmonton, Canada, Munich, Germany, and Christchurch, New Zealand show higher rates for women than men. Redrawn with permission from reference 10

be linked to sex steroids. Depressive symptoms may be noted more often during the premenstrual (late luteal) phase of the menstrual cycle. Depression is also more prevalent during the early postpartum period[11,12], perhaps due to declining levels of sex steroids. Although depression certainly occurs in the perimenopausal period, it is controversial whether the menopause represents a time of heightened psychiatric vulnerability[13,14]. When it does appear in association with the menopause, depression is more prevalent among those with a prior history of depression[15]. In addition, such menopausal symptoms as hot flushes, night sweats, insomnia, fatigue and dyspareunia clearly impact the quality of life[16]. Other psychological problems occurring during the perimenopausal period may increase vulnerability to depression. Stressful mid-life events include a husband's retirement, the 'empty nest' syndrome as adult children leave the home, or the burden of caring for ailing aged parents.

Older postmenopausal women who use estrogen typically report fewer depressive symptoms than non-users[17]. Beneficial effects of estrogen replacement on

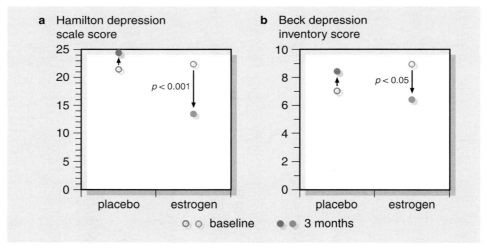

Figure 3.2. Estrogen and mood: results of two studies in asymptomatic women. (**a**) A total of 21 postmenopausal women (mean age 57 years) were randomized to placebo or estradiol valerate (2 mg/day) for 3 months. In the estrogen group, there was a significant decline ($p < 0.001$) between baseline and post-treatment scores on the Hamilton Depression Scale. Data are from reference 4. (**b**) A total of 36 women (mean age 53 years), who had undergone hysterectomy and oophorectomy, were randomly assigned to placebo or oral conjugated estrogens (1.25 mg/day (shown in the figure) or 0.625 mg/day (not shown)), administered 25 days per month for 3 months. In the two estrogen groups, there were significant declines ($p < 0.05$) between baseline and post-treatment scores on the Beck Depression Inventory. Data are from reference 7

mood are most often reported in healthy women without diagnosed depression or other psychopathology[5]. Among asymptomatic postmenopausal women in randomized trials of oral[4,7] or intramuscular[18] estrogen, active treatment reduced depressive scores, and hormone replacement had a substantial beneficial effect on the qualify of life[16,19] (Figure 3.2). No effect of estrogen on mood, however, is reported in other controlled studies[20].

Pharmacological potentiation of noradrenaline (norepinephrine) and serotonin are considered mainstays in the treatment of clinical depression. It is tempting to speculate that the estrogen effects on these monoaminergic neurotransmitter systems[21–27] are relevant to the clinical effects of estrogen on mood. The influence of estrogen might occur by several mechanisms, including the suppression of the activity of monoamine oxidase, a brain enzyme responsible for inactivation of both noradrenaline and serotonin[28]. Estrogen replacement is also known to increase blood levels of serotonin in postmenopausal women[29].

Estrogen has been infrequently evaluated in women suffering from major depression. One double-blind trial[30] found transdermal estradiol to be effective

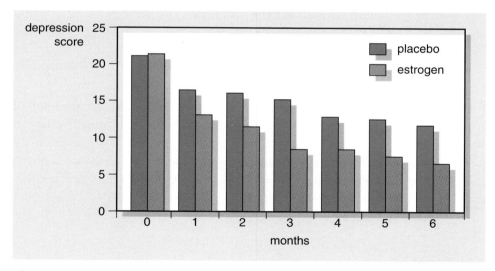

Figure 3.3. Effect of estrogen in postpartum depression. A total of 61 women (mean age 30 years) with severe postnatal depression were randomly assigned to placebo or active treatment (200 µg/day transdermal estradiol) for 6 months. After 3 months of unopposed estrogen, women in the active group were also given a progestogen for 12 days each month. Differences between the two treatment groups on the Edinburgh Postnatal Depression Scale were significant ($p < 0.001$). (On this scale, scores of at least 14 indicate major depression.) Data are from reference 30

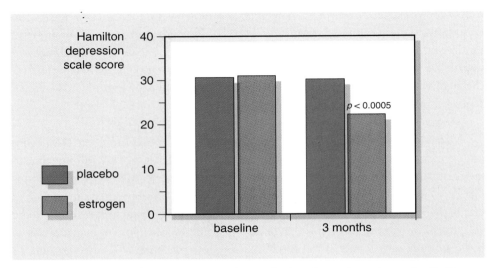

Figure 3.4. Effect of estrogen in major unipolar depression. A total of 40 pre-menopausal and postmenopausal women with Hamilton Depression Scale scores of at least 25 were randomly assigned to placebo or oral conjugated estrogens (up to 25 mg/day) for 3 months. For premenopausal women, estrogen was cycled with a progestogen; eight of 17 women in the placebo group, but only two of 23 women in the estrogen group, showed worse symptoms during the study. No one in the placebo group improved by 10 points on the Hamilton Depression Scale, whereas 11 women receiving estrogens improved by at least this amount. In the estrogen group, mean depression scores declined significantly ($p < 0.0005$). Data are from reference 31

for symptoms of severe postnatal depression (Figure 3.3). A second randomized study[31] used very high doses of oral conjugated estrogens in a 3-month study of women with severe unipolar depression. In this study, affective symptoms of women given active treatment abated significantly (Figure 3.4). Improvement was judged to be clinically meaningful, although residual depressive symptoms persisted in most study patients.

REFERENCES

1. Zweifel JE, O'Brien WH. A meta-analysis of the effect of hormone replacement therapy upon depressed mood. *Psychoneuroendocrinology* 1997;22:189–212

2. Ross JL, McCauley E, Roeltgen D, *et al.* Self-concept and behavior in adolescent girls with Turner syndrome: potential estrogen effects. *J Clin Endocrinol Metab* 1996;81:926–31

3. Hampson E. Estrogen-related variations in human spatial and articulatory–motor skills. *Psychoneuroendocrinology* 1990;15:97–111

4. Fedor-Freybergh P. The influence of oestrogens on the wellbeing and mental performance in climacteric and postmenopausal women. *Acta Obstet Gynecol Scand* 1977;Suppl 64:1–99

5. Schneider MA, Brotherton PL, Hailes J. The effect of exogenous oestrogens on depression in menopausal women. *Med J Aust* 1977;2:162–3

6. Sherwin BB. Affective changes with estrogen and androgen replacement therapy in surgically menopausal women. *J Affect Disord* 1988;14:177–87

7. Ditkoff EC, Crary WG, Cristo M, Lobo RA. Estrogen improves psychological function in asymptomatic postmenopausal women. *Obstet Gynecol* 1991;78:991–5

8. Best NR, Rees MP, Barlow DH, Cowen PJ. Effect of estradiol implant on noradrenergic function and mood in menopausal subjects. *Psychoneuroendocrinology* 1992;17:87–93

9. Montgomery JC, Appleby L, Brincat M, *et al.* Effect of oestrogen and testosterone implants on psychological disorders in the climacteric. *Lancet* 1987;1:297–9

10. Weissman MM, Bland R, Joyce RP, Newman S, Wells JE, Wittchen H-U. Sex differences in rates of depression: cross-national perspectives. *J Affect Disord* 1993;29:77–84

11. O'Hara MW, Zekoski EM, Philipps LH, Wright EJ. Controlled prospective study of post-partum mood disorders: comparison of childbearing and nonchildbearing women. *J Abnorm Psychol* 1990;99:3–15

12. Cox JL, Murray D, Chapman G. A controlled study of the onset, duration and prevalence of postnatal depression. *Br J Psychiatry* 1993;163:27–31

13. Ballinger CB. Psychiatric morbidity and the menopause; screening of the general population sample. *Br Med J* 1975;3:344–7

14. Hällström T, Samuelsson S. Mental health in the climacteric: the longitudinal study of women in Gothenburg. *Acta Obstet Gynecol Scand* 1985;Suppl 130:13–18

15. Hunter M. The South-East England longitudinal study of the climacteric and postmenopause. *Maturitas* 1992;14:117–26

16. Daly E, Gray A, Barlow D, McPherson K, Roche M, Vessey M. Measuring the impact of menopausal symptoms on quality of life. *Br Med J* 1993;307:836–40

17. Palinkas LA, Barrett-Connor E. Estrogen use and depressive symptoms in postmenopausal women. *Obstet Gynecol* 1992;80:30–6

18. Sherwin BB, Gelfand MM. Sex steroids and effect in the surgical menopause: a double-blind cross-over study. *Psychoneuroendocrinology* 1985;10:325–35

19. Limouzin-Lamothe M-A, Mairon N, Joyce CRB, Le Gal M. Quality of life after the menopause: influence of hormonal replacement therapy. *Am J Obstet Gynecol* 1994;170:618–24

20. Polo-Kantola P, Portin R, Polo O, Helenius H, Irjala K, Erkkola R. The effect of short-term estrogen replacement therapy on cognition: a randomized, double-blind, cross-over trial in postmenopausal women. *Obstet Gynecol* 1998;91:459–66

21. Greengrass PM, Tonge SR. The accumulation of noradrenaline and 5–hydroxytryptamine in three regions of mouse brain after tetrabenazine and iproniazid: effects of ethinyloestradiol and progesterone. *Psychopharmacologia* 1974;39:187–91

22. Ball P, Knuppen R, Haupt M, Breuer H. Interactions between estrogens and catechol amines. III. Studies on the methylation of catechol estrogens, catechol amines and other catechols by the catechol–O–methyltransferases of human liver. *J Clin Endocrinol Metab* 1972;34:736–46

23. Cohen IR, Wise PM. Effects of estradiol on the diurnal rhythm of serotonin activity in microdissected brain areas of ovariectomized rats. *Endocrinology* 1988;122:2619–25

24. Biegon A, Reches A, Snyder L, McEwen BS. Serotonergic and noradrenergic receptors in the rat brain: modulation by chronic exposure to ovarian hormones. *Life Sci* 1983;32: 2015–21

25. Sumner BEH, Fink G. Estrogen increases the density of 5-hydroxytryptamine$_{2A}$ receptors in cerebral cortex and nucleus accumbens in the female rat. *J Steroid Biochem Mol Biol* 1995;54:15–20

26. Fink G, Sumner BEH, Rosie R, Grace O, Quinn JP. Estrogen control of central neuro-transmission: effect on mood, mental state, and memory. *Cell Mol Neurobiol* 1996;16: 325–43

27. McQueen JK, Wilson H, Fink G. Estradiol-17β increases serotonin transporter (SERT) mRNA levels and the density of SERT-binding sites in female rat brain. *Mol Brain Res* 1997;45:13–23

28. Luine VN, McEwen BS. Effect of oestradiol on turnover of type A monoamine oxidase in brain. *J Neurochem* 1975;28:1221–7

29. Gonzales GF, Carrillo C. Blood serotonin levels in postmenopausal women: effects of age and serum oestradiol levels. *Maturitas* 1993;17:23–9

30. Gregoire AJP, Kumar R, Everitt B, Henderson AF, Studd JWW. Transdermal oestrogen for treatment of severe postnatal depression. *Lancet* 1996;347;930–3

31. Klaiber EL, Broverman DM, Vogel W, Kobayashi Y. Estrogen therapy for severe persistent depressions in women. *Arch Gen Psychiatry* 1979;36:550–4

4

Cognition

The term cognition encompasses the spectrum of intellectual abilities, including attention, learning and memory, language, perception, abstract reasoning and judgement. As reviewed below, there is accumulating evidence that estrogen may affect cognitive skills. However, even if one assumes the validity of positive findings, it is still important to consider whether the estrogen effects might be mediated indirectly. Both depression and anxiety can affect cognitive performance in older persons[1], and estrogen may modulate mood (see Chapter 3) and reduce stress[2,3]. It is likely that estrogen does influence cognitive skills independently of mood[4–6], but this caveat should be heeded in interpreting clinical data.

ANIMAL STUDIES

A number of studies of laboratory animals indicate that males outperform females on tasks of spatial memory. This male advantage appears to reflect the early organizational effects of sex steroids. For example, female neonatal rats treated with testosterone develop increased thickness of a portion of the hippocampus, and as adults these animals are better able to learn the location of a hidden platform submerged in a circular tank of water (water maze task)[7]. Sex differences in spatial learning may be mediated developmentally by the alpha estrogen receptor[8].

Estrogen enhances sensorimotor skills, such as those required to traverse a narrow beam[9], but behavioral data also indicate that estrogen influences learning and memory more directly (Figure 4.1). In one study, female rats learned to solve a water maze task less readily during the proestrus (high estrogen, high progesterone) phase of the estrous cycle than during diestrus[10]. However, a second study of spatial memory, which involved female rats that had undergone ovariectomy, found no effect of estrogen on a different maze task (radial maze)[11]. Ovariectomized rats administered estradiol performed somewhat better than control animals on a water-escape task, where animals were required to recall and choose the correct side of a two-choice water maze after a several minute delay[12]. In still

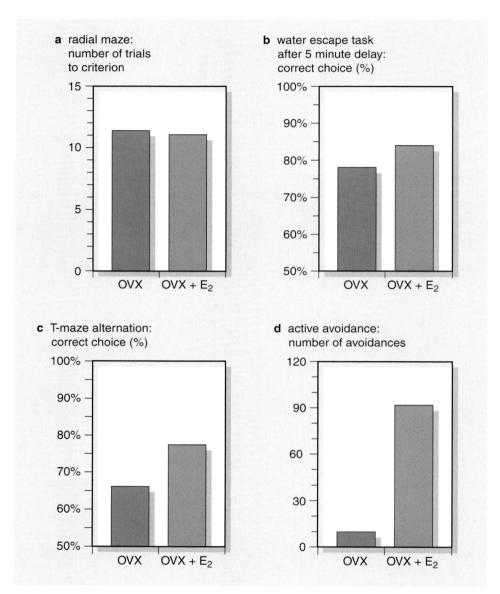

Figure 4.1. Estrogen and learning: four animal studies. After ovariectomy, young adult female rats were treated with placebo (OVX group) or estradiol (OVX + E$_2$). Partial results from four experiments are shown. A benefit of estrogen is suggested by results shown in (b), (c) and (d), but not (a). (**a**) Radial maze task. An animal was placed in the center of an eight-arm radial maze; a food receptacle was at the end of each arm. During a trial, an animal was allowed to visit arms in any order until all eight arms had been visited. The learning criterion was defined as five consecutive trials of at least seven correct choices (previously unentered arm) in the first eight visits; fewer trials to criterion represented better performance. Data are from reference 11. (**b**) Water escape task. To escape

another learning paradigm, estradiol significantly improved the performance of ovariectomized rats during acquisition of a task that required animals to alternate between two arms of a T-maze[13]. Finally, the performance of estrogen-treated ovariectomized rats was much better than that of control animals on an active avoidance task, in which animals learned to move from one side of a shuttle box to the other in order to avoid a foot shock[14].

HUMAN STUDIES

As with studies of laboratory animals, research with human subjects also suggests that estrogen is relevant to certain aspects of cognition. In women whose ovarian function was pharmacologically suppressed by leuprolide (a gonadotropin releasing hormone agonist), estrogen replacement altered the pattern of regional cerebral flow seen during an abstract reasoning task[15]. Regional blood flow in the cerebral cortex is an indirect marker of brain activation, and results of this experiment imply a role for estrogen in neural processes underlying cognition, although without clarifying what this role might be.

Estrogen effects on sundry cognitive measures have been examined in a plethora of clinical settings. One simple, and probably simplistic, interpretation of this body of human research is that estrogen maintains or enhances skills at which women tend to excel (for example, verbal abilities) but not skills conceptualized as male-advantaged (for example, visual–spatial abilities)[16]. A variation on this theme holds that estrogen particularly facilitates cognitive activities subserved to a greater

Figure 4.1. *continued*
from the water, an animal was allowed to swim to a submerged platform, whose location had been revealed 5 min previously. Two platform locations were possible in this water maze; chance level is 50%, and 100% represents perfect recall of the platform location. Data are from reference 12. (**c**) T-maze alternation task. On the first trial of each block, an animal received a food reward regardless of which arm of the two-arm T-maze was entered. On each of five subsequent trials, the animal was required to visit the arm not chosen on the previous trial to obtain a food reward. Data represent mean performance over 12 blocks of alternation trials, where chance performance is 50%. Data are from reference 13. (**d**) Active avoidance learning task. During each 1-min trial, a light and sound cue appeared, followed after a short delay by an electrical foot shock. Successful learning represented the avoidance of foot shock by transferring from one side of the shuttle box to the other after the onset of the cue and before the onset of the foot shock. Greater number of avoidances therefore represents better performance. Redrawn from reference 14

extent by the left than the right cerebral hemisphere[17]; verbal skills, of course, are acknowledged to be a left hemisphere function. Findings across studies, however, are not fully consistent, and any interpretation is complicated by the possibility that the cognitive effects of estrogen might well vary appreciably from one woman to the next[18].

During the follicular or luteal phase of the menstrual cycle, both characterized by high levels of estradiol, articulatory and motor skills are reported to be enhanced, and visuospatial skills impaired, compared to performances during the menstrual phase[16,19,20]. Other investigators found that information–processing speed[21], executive functions[22], non-verbal memory[23], or creativity[24] was relatively improved during high estrogen phases of the menstrual cycle. A few reports, however, indicated no discernible change in psychometric performance across the cycle[25].

Partially supportive evidence of an estrogen effect on cognition comes from an imaginative and intriguing study of trans-sexual men and women who were awaiting surgery for sex reassignment[26]. After baseline assessment, trans-sexual women were administered testosterone, while men received both an estrogen and an androgen antagonist. When results from both trans-sexual groups were considered together, findings implied a reciprocal relation between select verbal and visuospatial skills, which is mediated by sex steroids. Compared to baseline scores, testosterone given to female trans-sexuals was associated with improved visuospatial performance and impaired verbal fluency; in the estrogen plus anti-androgen male trans-sexual group, the trend was in the opposite direction (Figure 4.2).

Maternal plasma levels of estrogens are quite elevated during the course of pregnancy. Pregnant women sometimes rate their memory as worse than normal[27]. They may have more difficulty than control subjects with incidental (i.e. unintentional or unintended) learning[27], or they may recall information less well during the last trimester of pregnancy than during the postpartum period[28]. A decrement in the ability to perceive a simple figure embedded in a more complex drawing is also reported[29]. Complementing these human data, a preliminary report of age-matched nulliparous and multiparous rats suggested that multiparity enhances the ability to learn a spatial memory task[30]. The interpretation of these results in relation to endogenous estrogen exposure is problematic. In addition to estrogen elevations, pregnancy is associated with striking changes in serum levels of progesterone and other hormones. Undoubtedly, the dynamic interplay among complex physiological, psychological and social changes impacts the test perfor-

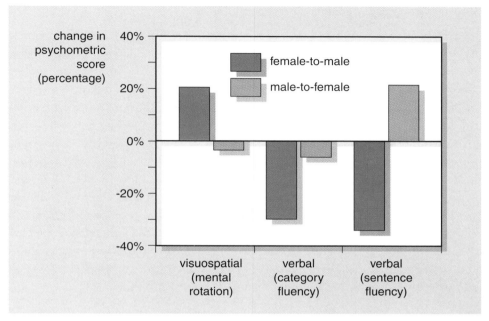

Figure 4.2. Change in cognitive scores after cross-sex hormonal therapy. Percentage change between baseline (pretreatment) scores and post-treatment scores among trans-sexual women (female-to-male, $n = 35$) given testosterone and trans-sexual men (male-to-female, $n = 15$) given ethinyl estradiol plus an antiandrogen (cyprotrone acetate). Visuospatial performance was assessed on a mental rotation task, and verbal performance was assessed on tasks of category and sentence fluency. Data are from reference 26

mance of pregnant women, and the specific contribution of estrogen has not yet been elucidated.

It is conceivable that some dietary estrogens may adversely affect certain aspects of cognition. Long-term behavioral deficits are reported in male rats which had nursed from mothers fed a diet high in the phytoestrogen coumes-trol[31]. Preliminary analyses from a cohort of Japanese-American women indicated that postmenopausal estrogen use was associated with better cognitive perform-ance, but this effect was apparent only among women reporting low dietary consumption of tofu (soybean curd)[32]. In a separate cohort of elderly Japanese-American men, a history of high levels of tofu consumption was associated with lower scores on a test of cognitive function[33].

Estrogen therapy and cognition: observational studies

Several small observational studies of healthy community-dwelling older women suggest that women who use hormone replacement (either unopposed estrogen, or estrogen plus a progestogen) may perform better on a broad spectrum of cognitive skills[5] or may outperform non-users on more discrete memory measures[34,35]. In a well-characterized aging cohort in Baltimore, women receiving estrogen performed significantly better than women who had never used estrogen on the Benton Visual Retention Test, a task that measures short-term non-verbal memory and drawing skills[36]. In this study, estrogen users seemed resistant to age-associated declines in test scores. A larger New York study found that older women who had used estrogen after the menopause scored better than women who had never used estrogen on tests of verbal memory, naming and abstract reasoning[37]. When women in this community-based cohort were retested several years later, mean scores on the verbal memory task had improved slightly among women who had previously used estrogen or were currently using estrogen, whereas scores of other women had declined slightly (Table 4.1).

A population-based case-control study from Austria found that postmenopausal women who were receiving estrogen performed better than non-users on

Table 4.1. Verbal memory score (mean ± SD) in a community-based cohort of older women (mean age 74 years) as a function of estrogen therapy. Comparisons are between women who had never used oral estrogen after the menopause and those who had used oral estrogen. Most women in the estrogen group were past users; all but 12 estrogen users had discontinued hormone therapy prior to testing. The immediate recall score on the Selective Reminding Test reflects the number of 12 unrelated words recalled after each of six learning trials. Delayed recall for these words was tested 15 min later. Data are from reference 37

	Estrogen never-users (n = 646)	Estrogen ever-users		
		All users (n = 81)	Users ≤ 1 year (n = 44)	Users > 1 year (n = 37)
Immediate recall (total of six trials)	39.8 ± 8.5	44.0 ± 8.8*	42.6 ± 8.9*	45.6 ± 8.5
Delayed recall	5.8 ± 2.3	6.7 ± 2.5*	6.4 ± 2.5	7.2 ± 2.5*

*$p < 0.05$, in comparison to never-users, after adjusting for age, education and ethnic group

a variety of psychometric tasks, most noticeably on tasks of complex problem solving and psychomotor speed[38]. In contrast, reports from two other large cohorts failed to identify appreciable differences on most cognitive measures when postmenopausal estrogen users were compared to non-users, although a subset of estrogen users in both of these cohorts performed better on measures of verbal fluency[39,40]. Other investigators found that serum estrogen levels measured in postmenopausal women did not predict subjects' performances on a clock-drawing task[41], on a brief cognitive screening instrument[42], or on timed tests of attention and psychomotor speed (the 'trails' task and the 'digit symbol' task)[42].

Estrogen therapy and cognition: randomized controlled trials

Compared to observational studies, randomized controlled trials can provide stronger evidence of an estrogen effect on cognition. An older report of women in a city residential facility for the aged compared estradiol injections (cycled with progesterone) to placebo injections[43]. After 6 months, the experimental group

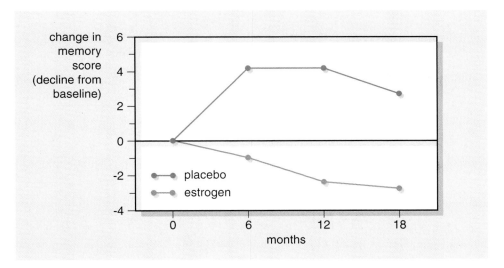

Figure 4.3. Estrogen and memory. Older women (mean age 75 years) in a home for the aged received intramuscular injections of placebo or estradiol benzoate (2 mg/week) with progesterone and testosterone. Mean changes from baseline scores on the Wechsler Memory Scale are shown for each group. Significant between-group differences in this randomized trial were observed at 6 and 12 months, but not at 18 months and not approximately 1 year after study termination (not shown). The number of participants declined from 28 to 21 during the 18 months of observation. Data are from reference 43

also received testosterone. During the 18-month trial, there was a tendency for treated women to improve slightly on a composite measure of verbal intelligence; group differences were significant at 12 months but not at 6 or 18 months[43]. On memory measures, differences favored the estrogen group at 6 and 12 months[43] (Figure 4.3). A second study of retirement-home residents used nurses' functional assessments of women given unopposed oral conjugated estrogens or placebo[44]. Over the 38-month observation period, women in the active treatment group were rated more favorably than other women (Figure 4.4). Weaknesses of both studies include a high dropout rate and the possibility that some subjects were cognitively impaired at baseline[43,44].

More recent placebo-controlled interventional trials of estrogen and cognition have better characterized their postmenopausal subjects. Several of these studies imply that women given estrogen outperform placebo-treated women on a variety of psychometric measures, including choice reaction time, attention and concentration, distractability, verbal memory and abstract reasoning[4,45,46]

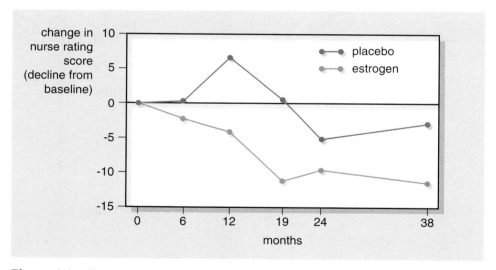

Figure 4.4. Estrogen and performance of daily activities. Women in a home for the aged (age range 60 to 91 years) were given placebo or oral conjugated estrogens (0.625 mg/day, 25 days per month) and rated by nurses on a questionnaire of interpersonal relations, self and social responsibility, and work and recreational activities. Women receiving estrogens showed less decline from baseline scores than women receiving placebo. The number of participants declined from 50 to 18 during the 38-month observation period. Redrawn from reference 44

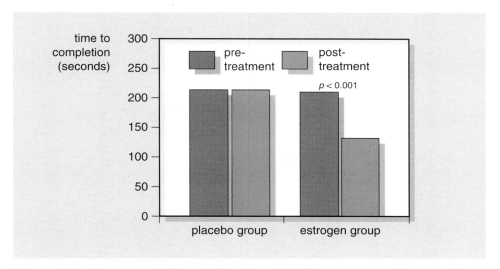

Figure 4.5. Estrogen and distractability. A total of 21 postmenopausal women (mean age 57 years) were randomized to oral estrogen (estradiol valerate 2 mg/day) versus placebo for 3 months. Women receiving active hormone were significantly faster in naming colors on the Stroop Color Interference Test. This timed task requires subjects to utter names of the ink color used to print 100 individual words, where each word is a color name printed in non-congruent color (e.g. the word 'red' printed in blue ink). Shorter times to complete the task suggest less distractability. Redrawn from reference 45

(Figure 4.5). Sherwin[4,6,46] has argued persuasively that estrogen-induced improvement is most apparent on tasks assessing the recall of verbal information, such as recalling details from a paragraph-length narrative. This contention is supported by her findings from healthy women with pharmacologically induced hypoestrogenism[6]. In this study, ovarian function was suppressed by a gonadotropin releasing hormone agonist. Three months later, when serum estradiol levels had declined to about a tenth of their pretreatment values, subjects scored lower on their recall of information from a paragraph narrative, compared to their baseline scores. Women were then randomly administered either estrogen or a placebo. When they were retested 2 months later, memory performance among women in the estrogen-treated group had returned to baseline but that of women in the placebo group remained depressed (Figure 4.6). In contrast to substantial effects on paragraph recall in this study, there were no significant differences across time on psychometric measures of short-term memory (digit span) or visual memory.

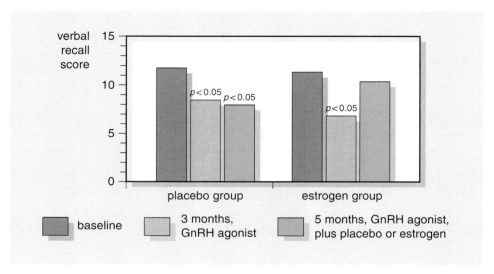

Figure 4.6. Estrogen and verbal recall. Ovarian function was suppressed in 19 women (mean age 35 years) with a gonadotropin releasing hormone (GnRH) agonist (leuprolide). After 3 months of treatment, subjects' ability to recall verbal information from a paragraph story after a 45 min delay was significantly impaired. In a randomized fashion, women then received a placebo or conjugated estrogens (0.625 mg/day). Two months later, recall was still impaired in the placebo group but not the estrogen group. Data are from reference 6

In general, the magnitude of an estrogen effect in healthy adults, when an effect is found, appears to be modest, but in some circumstances differences appear to be great enough to be clinically meaningful.

Despite the encouraging results summarized above, negative findings in another experimental trial are a cautionary reminder that much remains to be learned about estrogen effects on cognition. A randomized trial of 62 post-menopausal women (mean age 56 years) who had undergone a hysterectomy considered effects of transdermal estradiol versus placebo. Each treatment was given for 3 months in a cross-over design[47]. Psychometric measures focused on subjects' ability to process information rapidly (e.g. simple and choice reaction time tasks) and to sustain attention. Estrogen did not enhance performance on these particular tasks, and serum levels of estradiol failed to correlate with these particular psychometric scores.

REFERENCES

1. Deptula D, Singh R, Pomara N. Aging, emotional states, and memory. *Am J Psychiatry* 1993;150:429–34

2. Lindheim SR, Legro RS, Bernstein L, *et al*. Behavioral stress responses in premenopausal and postmenopausal women and the effects of estrogen. *Am J Obstet Gynecol* 1992;167: 1831–6

3. Del Rio G, Velardo A, Menozzi R, *et al*. Acute estradiol and progesterone administration reduced cardiovascular and catecholamine responses to mental stress in menopausal women. *Neuroendocrinology* 1998;67:269–74

4. Phillips SM, Sherwin BB. Effects of estrogen on memory function in surgically menopausal women. *Psychoneuroendocrinology* 1992;17:485–95

5. Kimura D. Estrogen replacement therapy may protect against intellectual decline in post-menopausal women. *Horm Behav* 1995;29:312–21

6. Sherwin BB, Tulandi T. 'Add-back' estrogen reverses cognitive deficits induced by a gonadotropin-releasing hormone agonist in women with leiomyomata uteri. *J Clin Endocrinol Metab* 1996;81:2545–9

7. Roof RL, Havens MD. Testosterone improves maze performance and induces development of male hippocampus in females. *Brain Res* 1992;572:310–13

8. Fugger HN, Cunningham SG, Rissman EF, Foster TC. Sex differences in the activational effect of ERα on spatial learning. *Horm Behav* 1998;34:163–70

9. Becker JB, Snyder PJ, Miller MM, Westgate SA, Jenuwine MJ. The influence of estrous cycle and intrastriatal estradiol on sensorimotor performance in the female rat. *Pharmacol Biochem Behav* 1987;27:53–9

10. Frye CA. Estrus-associated decrements in a water maze task are limited to acquisition. *Physiol Behav* 1994;57:5–14

11. Luine V, Rodriguez M. Effects of estradiol on radial arm maze performance of young and aged rats. *Behav Neural Biol* 1994;62:230–6

12. O'Neal MF, Means LW, Poole MC, Hamm RJ. Estrogen affects performance of ovariectomized rats in a two-choice water-escape working memory task. *Psychoneuroendocrinology* 1996;21:51–65

13. Fader AJ, Hendricson AW, Dohanich GP. Estrogen improves performance of reinforced T-maze alternation and prevents the amnestic effects of scopolamine administered systemically or intrahippocampally. *Neurobiol Learn Memory* 1998;69:225–40

14. Singh M, Meyer EM, Millard WJ, Simpkins JW. Ovarian steroid deprivation results in a reversible learning impairment and compromised cholinergic function in female Sprague–Dawley rats. *Brain Res* 1994;644:305–12

15. Berman KF, Schmidt PJ, Rubinow DR, *et al*. Modulation of cognition-specific cortical activity by gonadal steroids: a positron-emission tomography study in women. *Proc Natl Acad Sci USA* 1997;94:8836–41

16. Hampson E. Variations in sex-related cognitive abilities across the menstrual cycle. *Brain Cognit* 1990;14:26–43

17. Bibawi D, Cherry B, Hellige JB. Fluctuations of perceptual asymmetry across time in women and men: effects related to the menstrual cycle. *Neuropsychologia* 1995;33:131–8

18. Varney NR, Syrop C, Kubu CS, Struchen M, Hahn S, Franzen K. Neuropsychologic dysfunction in women following leuprolide acetate induction of hypoestrogenism. *J Assist Reproduct Genet* 1993;10:53–7

19. Hampson E, Kimura D. Reciprocal effects of hormonal fluctuations on human motor and perceptual-spatial skills. *Behav Neurosci* 1988;102:456–9

20. Hampson E. Estrogen-related variations in human spatial and articulatory-motor skills. *Psychoneuroendocrinology* 1990;15:97–111

21. Ho H-Z, Gilger JW, Brink TM. Effects of menstrual cycle on spatial information processes. *Percept Motor Skills* 1986;63:743–51

22. Keenan PA, Stern RA, Janowsky DS, Pedersen CA. Psychological aspects of premenstrual syndrome. I. Cognition and memory. *Psychoneuroendocrinology* 1992;17:179–87

23. Phillips SM, Sherwin BB. Variations in memory function and sex steroid hormones across the menstrual cycle. *Psychoneuroendocrinology* 1992;17:497–506

24. Krug R, Stamm U, Pietrowsky R, Fehm HL, Born J. Effects of menstrual cycle on creativity. *Psychoneuroendocrinology* 1994;19:21–31

25. Gordon HW, Lee PA. No difference in cognitive performance between phases of the menstrual cycle. *Psychoneuroendocrinology* 1993;18:521–31

26. Van Goozen SHM, Cohen-Kettenis PT, Gooren LJG, Frijda NH, Van de Poll NE. Gender differences in behaviour: activating effects of cross-sex hormones. *Psychoneuroendocrinology* 1995;20:343–63

27. Sharp K, Brindle PM, Brown MW, Turner GM. Memory loss during pregnancy. *Br J Obstet Gynaecol* 1993;100:209–15

28. Buckwalter JG, Stanczyk FZ, McCleary CA, *et al.* Pregnancy, the postpartum, and steroid hormones: effects on cognition and mood. *Psychoneuroendocrinology* 1999;24:69–84

29. Woodfield RL. Embedded figures test performance before and after childbirth. *Br J Psychol* 1984;75:81–8

30. Kinsley CH, Madonia L, Trainer R, *et al.* Motherhood enhances learning and memory: accompanying alterations in neuronal and glial morphology [abstr]. *Soc Neurosci Abstr* 1998;24:952

31. Whitten PL, Lewis C, Russell E, Naftolin F. Potential adverse effects of phytoestrogens. *J Nutr* 1995;125:771S–6S

32. Rice MM, Graves AB, Larson EB. Estrogen replacement therapy and cognition: role of phytoestrogens [abstr]. *Gerontologist* 1995;35(Suppl 1):169

33. White L, Petrovitch H, Ross GW, Masaki K. Association of mid-life consumption of tofu with late life cognitive impairment and dementia: the Honolulu–Asia Study [abstr]. *Neurobiol Aging* 1996;17(Suppl):S121

34. Robinson D, Friedman L, Marcus R, Tinklenberg J, Yesavage J. Estrogen replacement therapy and memory in older women. *J Am Geriatr Soc* 1994;42:919–22

35. Kampen DL, Sherwin BB. Estrogen use and verbal memory in healthy postmenopausal women. *Obstet Gynecol* 1994;83:979–83

36. Resnick SM, Metter EJ, Zonderman AB. Estrogen replacement therapy and longitudinal decline in visual memory. A possible protective effect? *Neurology* 1997;49:1491–7

37. Jacobs DM, Tang MX, Stern Y, *et al.* Cognitive function in nondemented older women who took estrogen after menopause. *Neurology* 1998;50:368–73

38. Schmidt R, Fazekas F, Reinhart B, *et al.* Estrogen replacement therapy in older women: a neuropsychological and brain MRI study. *J Am Geriatr Soc* 1996;44:1307–13

39. Szklo M, Cerhan J, Diez-Roux AV, *et al*. Estrogen replacement therapy and cognitive functioning in the Atherosclerosis Risk in Communities (ARIC) study. *Am J Epidemiol* 1996;144:1048–57

40. Barrett-Connor E, Kritz-Silverstein D. Estrogen replacement therapy and cognitive function in older women. *J Am Med Assoc* 1993;269:2637–41

41. Paganini-Hill A, Henderson VW. The effects of hormone replace therapy, lipoprotein cholesterol levels, and other factors on a clock drawing task in older women. *J Am Geriatr Soc* 1996;44:818–22

42. Yaffe K, Grady D, Pressman A, Cummings S. Serum estrogen levels, cognitive performance, and risk of cognitive decline in older community women. *J Am Geriatr Soc* 1998;46:816–21

43. Caldwell BM. An evaluation of psychological effects of sex hormone administration in aged women. II. Results of therapy after eighteen months. *J Gerontol* 1954;9:168–74

44. Kantor HI, Michael CM, Shore H. Estrogen for older women: a three-year study. *Am J Obstet Gynecol* 1973;116:115–18

45. Fedor-Freybergh P. The influence of oestrogens on the wellbeing and mental performance in climacteric and postmenopausal women. *Acta Obstet Gynecol Scand* 1977;Suppl 64:1–99

46. Sherwin BB. Estrogen and/or androgen replacement therapy and cognitive functioning in surgically menopausal women. *Psychoneuroendocrinology* 1988;13:345–57

47. Polo-Kantola P, Portin R, Polo O, Helenius H, Irjala K, Erkkola R. The effect of short-term estrogen replacement therapy on cognition: a randomized, double-blind, cross-over trial in postmenopausal women. *Obstet Gynecol* 1998;91:459–66

5
Dementia

The term dementia refers to the loss of mental, or cognitive, abilities severe enough to interfere substantially with one's usual daily activities. Dementia is not a specific diagnosis *per se*; dozens of different disorders diminish cognitive skills. Although dementia can develop at virtually any age, dementia is most characteristically a disorder of the elderly. Indeed, dementia is almost certainly the most feared accompaniment of aging.

Between the seventh and tenth decades of life, the prevalence of dementia doubles every 5 years[1]. The most common cause of dementia is Alzheimer's disease, accounting for about one-half to two-thirds of cases[2–4] (Figure 5.1). Dementia attributed to cerebrovascular disease, the second most prevalent cause, represents less than 10% of the total. Other disorders individually account for only small proportions of dementia cases.

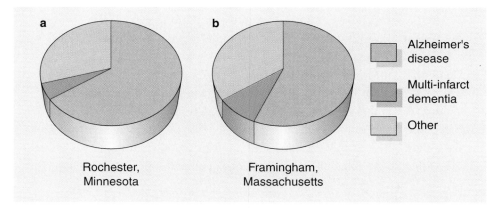

Figure 5.1. Causes of dementia. Incidence rates from Rochester, Minnesota (**a**) and prevalence rates from the Framingham, Massachusetts, cohort (**b**) indicate that Alzheimer's disease accounts for over half of the cases of dementia. Multi-infarct dementia, the next most common cause, accounts for fewer than a tenth of cases. Diagnoses in these two populations were based on clinical criteria, but autopsy-derived rates are similar[2]. Data are from references 3 and 4

ALZHEIMER'S DISEASE

The clinical diagnosis of Alzheimer's disease depends on the medical history, the absence of neurological signs implicating focal central nervous system disturbances, and laboratory tests that fail to indicate other illnesses that could lead to dementia[5] (Table 5.1). In Alzheimer's disease, dementia develops insidiously. The initial symptom often involves long-term episodic memory; i.e. there is an inability to learn and recall new events or newly presented information. Over time, there is a gradual but progressive loss of episodic memory and other cognitive skills, including difficulties with attention, naming, perception and abstract reasoning. Behavioral disturbances – for example, apathy, depression, suspiciousness, delusional thinking, or hallucinations – can occur but can be less prominent than in other dementing illnesses.

Pathological characteristics of Alzheimer's disease include neurofibrillary tangles within vulnerable neurons of the brain and neuritic plaques within the neuropil between nerve cell bodies[6,7] (Figure 5.2). Tangles are composed of

Table 5.1. Diagnostic criteria for Alzheimer's disease, adapted from reference 5

Clinically ascertained Alzheimer's disease ('probable Alzheimer's disease')
(1) Dementia
    (a) Cognitive deterioration affecting
        (i) episodic memory, plus
        (ii) at least one other area of cognitive functioning
    (b) Cognitive deterioration severe enough to interfere substantially with daily activities
(2) Dementia symptoms beginning in middle age or later
(3) Cognitive deficits not solely attributable to clouding of consciousness
(4) Gradual onset and progression of cognitive deficits
(5) Based on a thorough medical evaluation – one that includes neurological assessment, mental status testing, and appropriate laboratory tests – no other illness that could account for the patient's dementia

Pathologically verified Alzheimer's disease ('definite Alzheimer's disease')
(1) Dementia
(2) Neuropathological verification of numerous neuritic plaques in hippocampal and neocortical regions, usually accompanied by widespread neurofibrillary tangle formation in hippocampus and neocortex*

*More detailed pathological criteria are given in reference 6

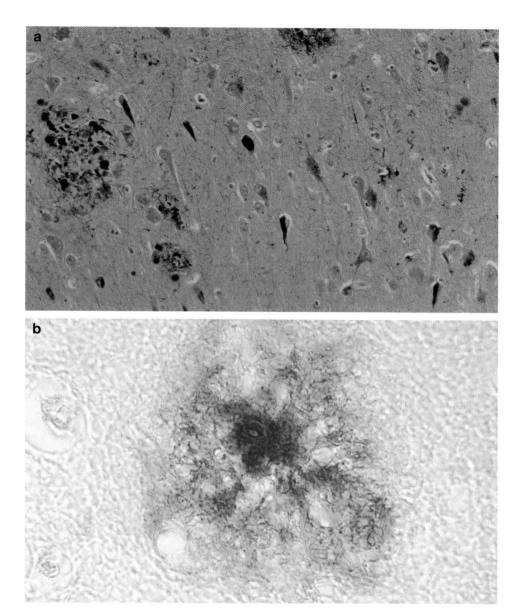

Figure 5.2. Pathology of Alzheimer's disease. (**a**) The silver-stained section of the hip-pocampus shows two key histopathological features of Alzheimer's disease: dark, flame-shaped intraneuronal neurofibrillary tangles and large globular neuritic plaques. Dystrophic neurites in the plaque appear as dark spheroids, whereas the central amyloid core is unstained in this preparation. (**b**) A neuritic plaque, shown in higher magnification than in (a), immunostained to reveal the amyloid core. Here, surrounding neurites are not visualized. Reproduced with permission from reference 7

paired helical filaments, which are derived from abnormal aggregates of tau protein. Tau is a microtubule-associated protein, which in Alzheimer's disease has been excessively phosphorylated. Plaques typically include dystrophic nerve processes (neurites), which also contain paired helical filaments, plus a central core of the β-amyloid polypeptide. The deposition of complement proteins, inflammatory cytokines and acute-phase reactants, as well as the presence of reactive astrocytes and microglia, suggests an inflammatory process[8,9] (Figure 5.3). Subsets of neurons are progressively isolated, as indicated by the severe pruning of their dendritic arborization[10] (Figure 5.4) and the loss of synaptic markers[11].

Some patients with Alzheimer's disease present in their 30s, 40s, or 50s. Disease in these rare early-onset cases is often inherited as an autosomal dominant disorder due to point mutations in identified genes. These genes encode two closely related presenilin proteins (chromosomes 14 and 1) and the amyloid precursor protein (chromosome 21)[12]. Our present understanding is that inheritance of one of these mutations almost inevitably culminates in symptoms of dementia by about age 60.

Late-onset Alzheimer's disease is more common and is not linked to autosomal dominant genetic mutations. The prevalence of Alzheimer's disease increases

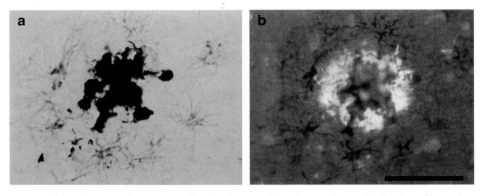

Figure 5.3. Photomicrograph of a single neuritic plaque from the brain of a patient with Alzheimer's disease, showing evidence of inflammation. (**a**) The figure on the left shows double-staining for a marker of microglia (human leukocyte antigen DR, purple) and astrocytes (glial fibrillary acidic protein, brown). Reactive microglia are seen within the plaque core which is ringed by reactive astrocytes. (**b**) The outline of the same plaque is shown on the right, where the β-amyloid core fluoresces as a pale yellow circle. Reproduced with permission from reference 9

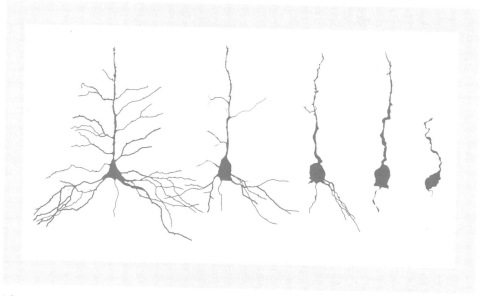

Figure 5.4. Loss of dendritic branches in Alzheimer's disease. As suggested by the left-to-right sequence in the figure, pyramidal neurons in the cerebral cortex undergo a progressive loss of dendritic branches at the time that a neurofibrillary tangle develops within the cell body. The figure is based on histological staining by the Golgi silver impregnation technique. Reproduced with permission from reference 10

exponentially with age[13] (Figure 5.5), and the illness is therefore most common among the oldest of the old. By some estimates, the prevalence approaches 50% after age 85 years[14]; other estimates are somewhat less ominous.

Although many genetic and environmental risk factors for late-onset disease remain to be identified, Alzheimer's risk is known to be strongly influenced by polymorphisms of apolipoprotein E[15], a glycoprotein involved in lipid transport and lipid metabolism. It is synthesized by astrocytes and microglia, as well as by other tissues. Within the brain, apolipoprotein E expression increases in the setting of neuronal injury, presumably reflecting lipid redistribution that occurs with the sprouting of nerve processes and the formation of new synapses[16,17]. A single genetic locus on the long arm of chromosome 19 encodes one of three common apolipoprotein E alleles. An elevated risk of Alzheimer's disease is associated with possession of the so-called ε4 allele[18], and the risk conferred by the ε4 allele is more evident among women than men[19,20].

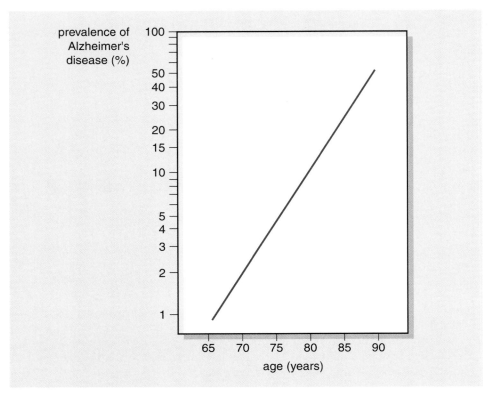

Figure 5.5. Prevalence of Alzheimer's disease as a function of age. The prevalence of dementia increases exponentially between ages 65 and 90 years, doubling about every 5 years. The graph is based on data from three studies, as summarized in reference 13

Gender is one of several factors postulated to influence development of late-onset Alzheimer's disease[21]. Most[19,22,23], but not all[24], observations indicate that the incidence of late-onset illness is greater for women than men. Alzheimer's disease is certainly more common in women (Table 5.2), due in part to their longer life expectancy and survival to late old age. Alzheimer's disease may also affect women differently than men. Women with Alzheimer's disease show greater deficits on semantic memory (naming) tasks than men[25,26] (Figure 5.6), but there is no evidence that overall severity differs between the sexes[27,28] (Figures 5.6 and 5.7).

Estrogen and Alzheimer's disease: possible mechanisms

There are a number of potential mechanisms by which estrogen deprivation after the menopause might influence the development or manifestations of Alzheimer's

Table 5.2. Prevalence of Alzheimer's disease, by sex, in various epidemiological studies. Adapted from reference 1. Other data suggest that the incidence, as well as the prevalence, of Alzheimer's disease may be greater for women than for men

Country or region	Number of studies	Ratio of female to male cases
Japan	4	1.9
Russia	1	3.5
Scandinavia	3	1.4
Britain	3	1.6
United States	2	3.0

Table 5.3. Estrogen actions potentially germane to Alzheimer's disease. Listed effects are not mutually exclusive. Adapted from reference 29

Effects on neuronal growth and synaptic plasticity
Modulation of neurotrophin action
Effects on neurotransmitter systems, including
   acetylcholine
   norepinephrine
   serotonin
   others (dopamine, γ-aminobutyric acid, glutamate, opioid peptides)
Diminished programmed cell death (apoptosis)
Increased brain expression of apolipoprotein E
Induction of tau protein
Reduced formation of β-amyloid
Reduced inflammation
Antioxidant properties
Blunting of the stress response
Augmentation of cerebral blood flow
Enhanced cerebral metabolism

disease[29] (Tables 2.3 and 5.2). Cell bodies of origin for widely projecting subcortical and brain stem nuclei are heavily affected by neurofibrillary tangle formation in Alzheimer's disease. These nuclei supply cholinergic, noradrenergic and serotonergic input to other brain regions, and these neurotransmitter systems are among those influenced by estrogen[30–32]. The effects of estrogen on basal forebrain cholinergic neurons appear especially important in relation to Alzheimer's

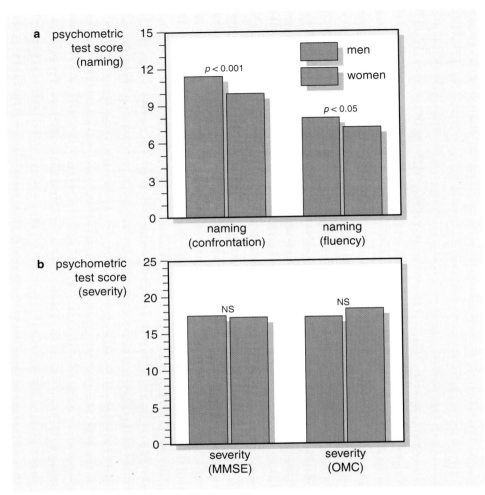

Figure 5.6. Naming skills of men and women with Alzheimer's disease. (a) When men ($n = 270$) and women ($n = 377$) with Alzheimer's disease were compared, men performed significantly better on semantic memory (naming) tasks than women, but there were no significant differences on measures of global severity (b). Analyses were adjusted for age, education and duration of dementia symptoms. For naming, mean scores on a 15-item confrontation (picture) naming task and a 60-s category naming (fluency) task are shown. Severity scores are from the Mini-Mental State examination (MMSE; maximum score [best] 30) and the Orientation–Memory–Concentration test (OMC; maximum error score [worst] 28). NS, not significant. Data are from reference 26

disease. It is known that cholinergic blockade impedes episodic memory[33], and basal forebrain pathology in Alzheimer's disease contributes to cognitive deficits[34].

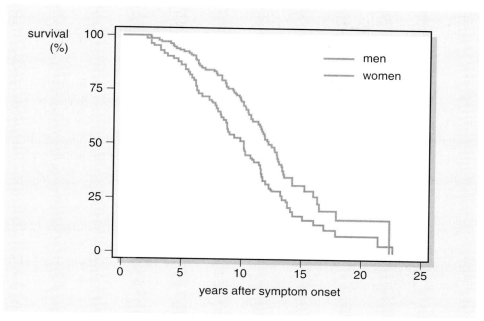

Figure 5.7. Survival in Alzheimer's disease, by sex. Survival from onset of dementia symptoms to death in patients with Alzheimer's disease. In this voluntary cohort, the average age at symptom onset was 67.4 years for men ($n = 98$) and 69.3 years for women ($n = 151$). The median survival was significantly greater for women (12.8 years) than for men (10.2 years). Slightly longer survival for women is consistent with the fact that women generally live longer than men. In the context of Alzheimer's disease, this finding implies that Alzheimer's severity, as inferred from survival data, is similar for men and women. Data are from reference 23

In adult female rats, ovariectomy reduces, and estrogen replacement increases, cholinergic markers in the basal forebrain and in projection target areas[35–38]. Estrogen may protect against programmed cell death (apoptosis)[39] implicated in Alzheimer's disease.

The interactions of estrogen with neurotrophins may also be important. Neurotrophins are proteins that are important for the maintenance of neuronal viability and for the promotion of neuronal growth and differentiation. Two of the neurotrophins, nerve growth factor and brain-derived neurotrophic factor, help maintain the viability of cholinergic neurons after experimental lesions[40,41], and some have advocated nerve growth factor for the treatment of Alzheimer's symptoms[42]. Basal forebrain cholinergic neurons possess receptors for both estrogen and neurotrophins, and estrogen may modulate the effects of neuro-trophin in this region[43,44], for example, through up–regulating the expression of the receptor for nerve growth factor[45].

Estrogen influences two key proteins implicated in Alzheimer's disease patho-logy: tau and β–amyloid. Estrogen induces tau formation, a process that coincides with enhanced growth of axons and dendrites[46]. Estrogen also acts to reduce the formation of β–amyloid. The large amyloid precursor protein, encoded by a normal chromosome 21 gene, can be proteolytically processed at alternative sites. At physiological concentrations, estradiol leads to degradation products unable to accumulate as β–amyloid[47].

Several observations imply an important link between estrogens and apolipoprotein E. In the serum, estrogen reduces apolipoprotein E levels[48], but in some brain regions estrogen acts to increase the expression of apolipoprotein E[49] (Figure 5.8). Experimental lesions that disrupt cholinergic input to the hippo-campus elevate apolipoprotein E in denervated areas[50], and estrogen–induced sprouting to these areas requires apolipoprotein E[51]. In Alzheimer's disease, cholinergic deficits are not associated with an increase in apolipoprotein E protein levels; on the contrary, levels are reduced both in cerebrospinal fluid[52] and in the hippocampus[53]. Interestingly, hippocampal reductions of apolipoprotein E are greater for ε4 homozygotes than for other apolipoprotein E genotypes[53]. Speculatively, estrogen replacement could facilitate neuronal repair in Alzheimer's disease by increasing apolipoprotein E expression in the brain.

Other estrogen properties might protect brain function in patients with Alzheimer's disease. These include effects on inflammation, free radicals and cortisol. Inflammatory responses are implicated in neuritic plaque formation[8,54], and estrogen may moderate some aspects of the inflammatory process[55,56] . Free radicals accumulate with aging, and these highly reactive molecules damage lipids, proteins and nucleic acids. Oxidative damage is prominent in the brains of Alzheimer's patients[57]. The toxicity of β–amyloid may be mediated or potentiated by free radicals[58,59]. At physiological concentrations, estrogens act as anti-oxidants[60–62], with different estrogens possessing different antioxidant properties (Figure 5.9).

Estrogen replacement therapy in postmenopausal women blunts cortisol eleva-tions that are induced by psychological or physical stress[63]. As a reflection of hypothalamic–pituitary–adrenal reactivity, baseline cortisol levels are elevated in Alzheimer's disease[64], and in Alzheimer's patients there is an association between

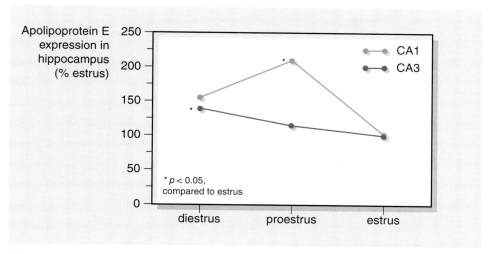

Figure 5.8. Estrogen and apolipoprotein E expression in the brain. In the CA1 region of the hippocampus, but not the CA3 region, the number of synapses fluctuates during the rat estrous cycle; there are more synapses during proestrus when estrogen levels are rising than during estrus when levels are low. Apolipoprotein E is produced by glial cells in the brain. As shown above, the expression of apolipoprotein E messenger RNA (grain density per cell in *in situ* hybridization experiments) increases during proestrus in the CA1 but not the CA3 region; in the CA3 region, apolipoprotein E expression was higher during diestrus. Proestrus versus estrus differences were also found in the arcuate nucleus of the hypothalamus (not shown), another brain area where synapse number is greater during proestrus. Data are from reference 49

dementia severity and both hypothalamic–pituitary–adrenal reactivity[65] and atrophy of hippocampal structures[66]. Stress impairs memory[67] and experimental stress can lead to neuronal atrophy or cell death within the hippocampus[68]. It is thus possible that estrogen could enhance memory through moderating the deleterious effects of stress (Figure 5.10).

Estrogen actions are multifaceted and the magnitude of a given neurotrophic or neuroprotective effect often varies among different estrogens. Indeed, it is possible that some estrogenic compounds adversely affect the risk of Alzheimer's disease. For example, a high level of dietary tofu consumption was associated with an increased risk of Alzheimer's disease in a large cohort of elderly Japanese-American men[69]. Speculatively, such a finding could result if the phytoestrogens in tofu functioned as antiestrogens at the receptor level or acted as competitive or non-competitive inhibitors of other estrogenic compounds.

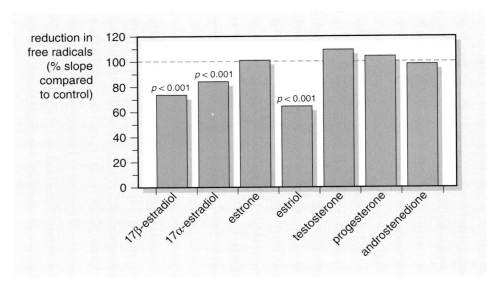

Figure 5.9. Antioxidant effect of estrogens and other steroids. Antioxidant effects were assayed using a phycoerythrin fluorescence assay, in which fluorescent decay was induced by a free radical generator. The slope of the fluorescence decay curve in the presence of hormone is expressed as a percentage of the slope in the absence of hormone. In this assay, the strongest antioxidant effects were shown by estriol and 17β-estradiol. Data are from reference 61

Estrogen therapy and risk of Alzheimer's disease

The possibility that pharmacological estrogen replacement after the menopause might protect against Alzheimer's disease has been examined in a number of epidemiological studies. In considering these reports, however, it is important to acknowledge that women who use estrogen differ from those who do not[70,71], and bias or unrecognized confounding cannot be fully excluded in some observational analyses.

Several early case–control studies that explored estrogen usage as one of a number of potential risk factors for Alzheimer's disease failed to discern a significant association with Alzheimer's risk. The number of estrogen users in these studies was small, however, limiting the power to detect a possible association. A 1994 analysis of volunteers in a longitudinal study of aging and dementia found current estrogen use to be significantly more common among elderly non-demented women than among age-equivalent women diagnosed with Alzheimer's disease[25]. In this study, cases and controls did not differ with respect to total numbers of prescription medications or prior gynecological procedures

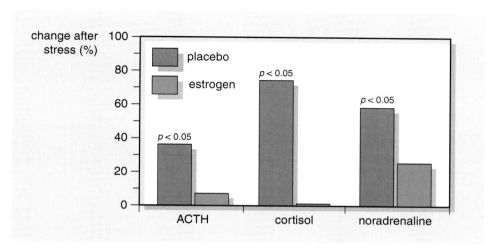

Figure 5.10. Effect of estrogen on psychological stress. A total of 36 postmenopausal women were randomly assigned to receive placebo or transdermal estrogen (0.1 mg estradiol) for 6 weeks. Stress was then induced by psychological tasks or the cold pressor test. The figure shows maximum percentage changes, compared to baseline serum levels, in adrenocorticotropic hormone (ACTH), cortisol and noradrenaline. Significant elevations in these markers of stress reactivity occurred only in the placebo group. Redrawn with permission from reference 63

that might have influenced the use of hormone therapy. Other subsequently reported analyses based on current hormone use[72,73] or derived from data on hormone use that were obtained retrospectively[74,75] also implied that estrogen is protective (Figure 5.11).

Notable weaknesses mar interpretation of these cross-sectional studies. If women with cognitive symptoms were less likely to be prescribed hormone replacement, the resultant bias would overestimate the association favoring the hypothesis that estrogen is protective. Conversely, the association could be underestimated if estrogen prescriptions were more likely to be given to cognitively impaired women. Moreover, bias could have been introduced when information on estrogen use was often obtained differently from a demented case (asking a family member or other surrogate informant for this information) than from a healthy control (asking the woman herself).

Recent case–control and cohort studies provide stronger evidence for a protective effect of estrogen. In some of these analyses, estrogen use was documented

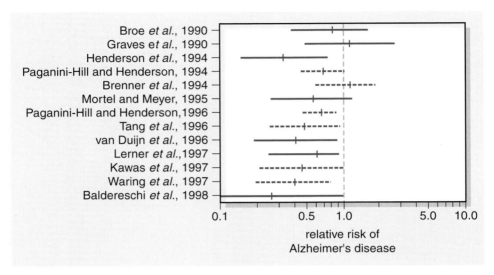

Figure 5.11. Estrogen replacement therapy and Alzheimer's disease risk. Point estimates of relative risk and 95% confidence intervals are shown for case–control and cohort studies published since 1990. Estimates less than one indicate a protective effect. Studies in which information on estrogen use was collected prospectively (indicated by stippled bars) are the Seattle study of Brenner and colleagues[77], the Leisure World studies of Paganini-Hill and Henderson[76,79] (cases in these two studies were not independent of each other), the New York study of Tang and colleagues[78], the Baltimore Longitudinal Study of Kawas and colleagues[80] and the Rochester, Minnesota, study of Waring and colleagues[81]

prospectively, before some women developed symptoms of dementia[76–81] (Figure 5.11). The largest such study is from the Leisure World retirement community cohort in southern California[79]. In this nested case–control study, 248 cases of Alzheimer's disease were identified on the basis of death certificate records and were matched with 1198 controls whose death certificates did not indicate dementia. Forty-eight per cent of controls but only 39% of cases had used estrogen after the menopause, and estrogen users had a 35% lower risk of Alzheimer's disease. Similar risk reductions were found when analyses in this cohort were restricted to oral estrogen use. Although Alzheimer's disease is almost certainly under-reported on death certificate records, the effect of these missing cases would be to reduce the magnitude of any association rather than to suggest an association in the absence of any true effect on Alzheimer's risk.

Protective effects are also reported in analyses from New York[78], Baltimore[80], and Rochester, Minnesota[81], where estrogen users had risk reductions of about one-half. In the New York City cohort, protective effects were evident for women with the ε4 apolipoprotein E allele and women without this allele. Moreover, the age when dementia was first diagnosed was later in women who had taken estrogen than in women who had never used hormone replacement.

Not all studies document an association between estrogen and Alzheimer's disease, however. In a health maintenance organization population in Seattle, Washington, computerized pharmacy records were examined for women who had developed Alzheimer's disease and for matched controls without dementia[77]. About half of women in both groups had filed at least one prescription for estrogen. As in the Leisure World cohort, the risk of an Alzheimer diagnosis was reduced by nearly a third among women who had previously used oral estrogens, but here the reduction was not statistically significant and no protective effect at all was evident when all types of estrogen preparations were considered.

Estrogen replacement and Alzheimer's risk: strength of association

If estrogen reduces the risk of Alzheimer's disease, then it might be expected that greater estrogen exposure would be more protective than lesser exposure. Consistent with this prediction, a significant dose effect was observed in the Leisure World study[76,79]. Here, the risk of Alzheimer's disease decreased significantly with higher dosages of the most often prescribed oral estrogen (Figure 5.12). Similarly, increasing duration of postmenopausal estrogen use was associated with greater risk reductions in both the Leisure World[76,79] and the New York[78] studies (Figure 5.13), and in the Rochester study risk estimates among estrogen-users decreased with increasing duration of estrogen use and with increasing cumulative estrogen dose[81]. In the Baltimore study[80], however, the duration of estrogen use did not influence risk estimates.

Estrogen therapy and cognitive deficits of Alzheimer's disease

Women with Alzheimer's disease taking estrogen perform better on a variety of cognitive tasks than women with Alzheimer's disease who are not taking estrogen[25,82] (Figure 5.14). In one study, differences favoring estrogen users were more apparent on the ability to provide word names[82], a task that is relatively more difficult for women with Alzheimer's disease than it is for men with this diagnosis[26,27] (Figure 5.6).

Recent intervention trials have examined estrogen effects in women with Alzheimer's disease, although only a few reports provide full details[83–88]. Sample

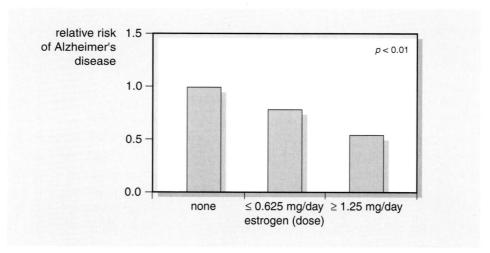

Figure 5.12. Estrogen replacement therapy and Alzheimer's disease risk: effect of dosage. In the Leisure World cohort[77], the most common estrogen preparation was conjugated estrogens. When the longest-used oral dosage was considered, women who used higher doses (≥ 1.25 mg/day) had a lower risk of Alzheimer's disease than women using lower doses (≤ 0.625 mg/day). The reference dosage is none (relative risk = 1). The trend between increasing dose and lower risk was significant ($p < 0.01$)

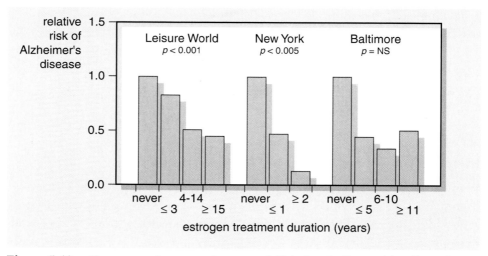

Figure 5.13. Estrogen replacement therapy and Alzheimer's disease risk: effect of treatment duration. In the Leisure World[77] and New York[76] studies, but not the Baltimore study[78], there was a significant relationship between increasing duration of estrogen use and lower risk of Alzheimer's disease. The reference group consists of never-users (relative risk = 1). NS, not significant

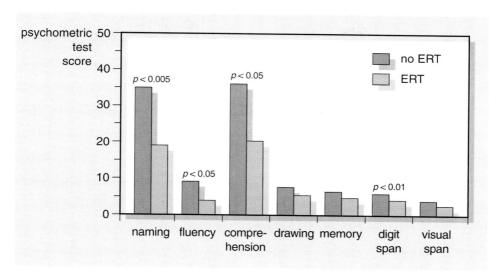

Figure 5.14. Estrogen replacement and psychometric performance in Alzheimer's disease. In this observational study, nine women with Alzheimer's disease currently using estrogen replacement therapy (ERT) were matched to 27 women with Alzheimer's disease not using estrogen. Matching criteria were age, education and duration of dementia symptoms. Compared to non-users, estrogen users performed somewhat better on several psychometric measures, with the largest differences being on the confrontation naming task. Data are from reference 82

sizes have been small, and overall results must be considered cautiously[89]. Only two of these studies followed women for longer than 6 weeks[86,88], and most trials have been conducted as open-label studies. One randomized trial of estrogen in Alzheimer's disease has been fully reported. In this short-term Japanese study[85], women with Alzheimer's disease received either oral conjugated estrogens or placebo. After 3 weeks of treatment, women in the active arm improved significantly over baseline on each of three brief psychometric measures (Figure 5.15). Preliminary findings in two other randomized trials are also encouraging[90,91].

Some of the postulated estrogen effects in women with Alzheimer's disease may be mediated through interactions with cholinergic neurons. This contention is supported by studies of ovariectomized rats required to alternate between the two arms of a T-maze[92,93]. After the administration of scopolamine (a high-affinity blocker of the cholinergic muscarinic receptor), maze performance deteriorated. However, deleterious effects of scopolamine were reversed by estrogen replacement. Complementary findings were reported on a water-maze task,

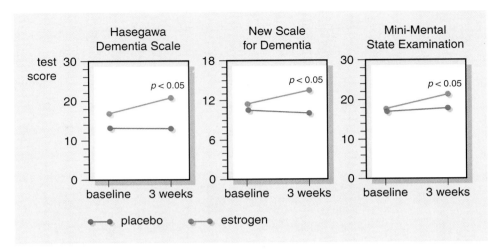

Figure 5.15. Effects of estrogen on cognitive performance in Alzheimer's disease. Women with Alzheimer's disease ($n = 14$, mean age 84 years) were randomly assigned to receive placebo or 1.25 mg/day of conjugated estrogens. After 3 weeks, estrogen users had improved significantly over baseline on the revised version of the Hasegawa Dementia Scale, the New Scale for Dementia and the Mini-Mental State Examination. Women in the placebo group did not show significant changes. Redrawn with permission from reference 85

where estrogen enhancement of learning was blocked by scopolamine[94]. In Alzheimer's disease, drugs that inhibit acetylcholinesterase (e.g. tacrine and donepezil) act to increase brain levels of acetylcholine and are of modest therapeutic benefit[95,96]. In a retrospective analysis of data from a multicenter cholinesterase inhibitor trial in patients with Alzheimer's disease, women using hormone replacement at the time of study enrollment and subsequently randomized to receive the anticholinesterase agent performed significantly better than women randomized to the placebo arm[97]. Performance of demented women in the active treatment arm who were not using estrogen was similar to that of women in the placebo group (Figure 5.16). Findings must be interpreted cautiously, however, as estrogen use in this study was not randomized, and the number of women using hormone replacement was small.

No large placebo-controlled, double-blind trial of estrogen has been conducted over a substantial time period, although such trials are currently under way. Conclusions regarding estrogen and Alzheimer's symptoms are therefore not yet possible despite promising results from smaller trials[89]. Moreover, limited

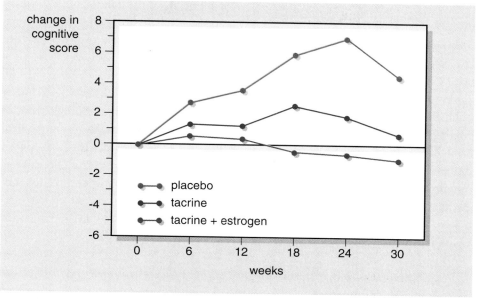

Figure 5.16. Change in cognitive performance in Alzheimer's disease: effect of estrogen plus a cholinergic agent. Post hoc analyses of a randomized trial of an acetylcholinesterase inhibitor (tacrine) subdivided women in the active treatment arm into those who were receiving estrogen ($n = 8$) and those not receiving hormone replacement ($n = 50$). On the cognitive subscale of the Alzheimer's Disease Assessment Scale, women receiving tacrine plus estrogen improved significantly over baseline scores ($p = 0.02$) and improved significantly when compared to women ($n = 50$) in the placebo group not receiving estrogen ($p = 0.009$). Performances of women in the placebo group and non-estrogen users in the tacrine group did not change significantly during this 30-week trial. Redrawn with permission from reference 97

data imply that there is less likely to be a role for estrogen among women whose dementia is relatively severe[83,98]. Progesterone can potentiate, as well as down-regulate, the neurotrophic effects of estrogen[99,100], and preliminary observations raise the concern that putative estrogen benefits in Alzheimer's disease would be attenuated when a progestogen is included in the hormone regimen[88,97].

Indirect markers of estrogen exposure

After the menopause, estrogen production is derived largely through the aromatization of androstenedione to estradiol. Androstenedione and its precursor dehydroepiandrosterone are produced by stroma cells of the ovary and by cells in the inner zone of the adrenal cortex. Conversion to estrogen occurs in peripheral sites, notably adipose tissue. Among older women, body weight is therefore correlated with circulating levels of estrogen[101]. Moreover, greater weight is associated with lower levels of sex hormone binding globulin[102], thus increasing the availability of free estrogen. Alzheimer's patients tend to be thinner than other older persons[103], and, speculatively, body weight might modify a woman's risk of Alzheimer's disease. Among women in the population-based Italian Longitudinal Study on Aging[75], estimated weight at age 50 was not associated with Alzheimer's disease. In the Leisure World study, however, higher body weight at the time of initial cohort enrollment was associated with a reduced likelihood of a subsequent Alzheimer's disease diagnosis[79]. For women who weighed at least 63 kg the estimated risk of developing Alzheimer's disease was about 30% lower than for women who weighed less than 56 kg.

Among women with Alzheimer's disease, body weight is also associated with scores on tests of cognitive skills. An analysis of psychometric scores from a large convenience sample of women with this diagnosis demonstrated a significant association between greater weight and better performance on two cognitive tasks (the Mini-Mental State examination and the cognitive subscore of the Alzheimer's Disease Assessment Scale); these analyses were adjusted for height, symptom duration, age and education[104]. When two weight extremes (40 versus 80 kg) were considered, it was calculated that weight differences could account for performance differences on the two tasks of about 12 and 20%, respectively[104].

Exposures to endogenous sex steroids might modify disease risk, when the disease in question is hormonally sensitive. In this regard, investigators have considered early age at menarche, late age at menopause and increased parity as factors that might reduce Alzheimer's risk. Earlier age at menarche was associated with a significantly lower risk of Alzheimer's disease in the Italian Longitudinal Study on Aging[75], and a similar trend was reported from Leisure World[79]. However, in these two cohorts[75,79], as well as in another well-characterized cohort of predominately late-onset Alzheimer's cases[78], the predicted association with later age at menopause was not observed. In contrast, a European study of early-onset familial cases found an association between younger age at menopause and increased Alzheimer's risk[105]. In the Leisure World study and the Italian Longitudinal Study, parity was unrelated to the risk of Alzheimer's disease[75,79].

VASCULAR DEMENTIA

It remains controversial whether estrogen replacement affects the incidence of stroke (see Chapter 6). Even greater uncertainty exists regarding potential estrogen effects on dementia attributed to cerebrovascular disease, which in its most common form is referred to as multi-infarct dementia. One case–control study compared 65 women with a clinical diagnosis of vascular dementia with 148 older women without dementia[73]. In analyses based on current estrogen use, demented patients were less likely to be receiving hormone therapy than controls, but differences were not statistically significant. Resolution of this controversial issue will come only with additional data from well-designed cohort studies and randomized primary prevention trials of estrogen.

REFERENCES

1. Jorm AF, Korten AE, Henderson AS. The prevalence of dementia: a quantitative integration of the literature. *Acta Psychiatr Scand* 1987;76:465–79
2. Kokmen E, Offord KP, Okazaki H. A clinical and autopsy study of dementia in Olmstead County, Minnesota, 1980–1981. *Neurology* 1987;37:426–30
3. Schoenberg BS, Kokmen E, Okazaki H. Alzheimer's disease and other dementing illnesses in a defined United States population: incidence rates and clinical features. *Ann Neurol* 1987;22:724–9
4. Bachman DL, Wolf PA, Linn R, *et al.* Prevalence of dementia and probable senile dementia of the Alzheimer type in the Framingham Study. *Neurology* 1992;42:115–9
5. McKhann G, Drachman D, Folstein MF, Katzman R, Price D, Stadlan EM. Clinical diagnosis of Alzheimer's disease: report of the NINCDS-ADRDA Work Group under the auspices of Department of Health and Human Services Task Force on Alzheimer's Disease. *Neurology* 1984;34:939–44
6. Mirra SS, Heyman A, McKeel D, *et al.* Consortium to Establish a Registry for Alzheimer's Disease (CERAD). Part II. Standardization of the neuropathologic assessment of Alzheimer's disease. *Neurology* 1991;41: 479–86
7. Iqbal K, Grundke-Iqbal I. Neurofibrillary degeneration. In de Leon MJ, ed. *An Atlas of Alzheimer's Disease.* Carnforth, UK: Parthenon Publishing, 1999
8. McGeer PL, McGeer EG. The inflammatory response system of brain: implications for therapy of Alzheimer and other neurodegenerative diseases. *Brain Res Rev* 1995;21: 195–218
9. Itagaki S, McGeer PL, Akiyama H, Zhu S, Selkoe D. Relationship of microglia and astrocytes to amyloid deposits of Alzheimer's disease. *J Neuroimmunol* 1989;24:173–82
10. Scheibel ME, Lindsay RD, Tomiyasu U, Scheibel AN. Progressive dendritic changes in aging human cortex. *Exp Neurol* 1975;47:392–403
11. Alford MF, Masliah E, Hansen LA, Terry RD. A simple dot-immunobinding assay for quantification of synaptophysin-like immunoreactivity in human brain. *J Histochem Cytochem* 1994;42:283–7

12. Pericak-Vance MA, Haines JL. Genetic susceptibility to Alzheimer disease. *Trends Genet* 1995;11:504–18

13. Katzman R. Education and the prevalence of dementia and Alzheimer's disease. *Neurology* 1993;43:13–20

14. Evans DA, Funkenstein HH, Albert MS, *et al.* Prevalence of Alzheimer's disease in a community population of older persons: higher than previously reported. *J Am Med Assoc* 1989;262:2551–6

15. Strittmatter WJ, Saunders AM, Schmechel D, *et al.* Apolipoprotein E: high-avidity binding to β-amyloid and increased frequency of type 4 allele in late-onset familial Alzheimer disease. *Proc Natl Acad Sci USA* 1993;90:1977–81

16. Mahley RW. Apolipoprotein E: cholesterol transport protein with expanding role in cell biology. *Science* 1988;240:622–30

17. Poirier J. Apolipoprotein E in animal models of CNS injury and in Alzheimer's disease. *Trends Neurosci* 1994;17:525–30

18. Seshadri S, Drachman DA, Lippa CF. Apolipoprotein E ε4 allele and the lifetime risk of Alzheimer's disease. *Arch Neurol* 1995;52:1074–9

19. Payami H, Zareparsi S, Montee KR, *et al.* Gender difference in apolipoprotein E-associated risk for familial Alzheimer disease: a possible clue to the higher incidence of Alzheimer disease in women. *Am J Hum Genet* 1996;58:803–11

20. Poirier J, Davignon J, Bouthillier D, Kogan S, Bertrand P, Gauthier S. Apolipoprotein E polymorphism and Alzheimer's disease. *Lancet* 1993;342:697–9

21. Graves AB, Kukull WA. The epidemiology of dementia. In Morris JC, ed. *Handbook of Dementing Illnesses.* New York: Marcel Dekker, 1994:23–69

22. Katzman R, Aronson M, Fuld P, *et al.* Development of dementing illnesses in an 80-year-old volunteer cohort. *Ann Neurol* 1989;25:317–24

23. Fratiglioni L, Viitanen M, von Strauss E, Tontodonati V, Herlitz A, Winblad B. Very old women at highest risk of dementia and Alzheimer's disease: incidence data from the Kungsholmen Project, Stockholm. *Neurology* 1997;48:132–8

24. Bachman DL, Wolf PA, Linn RT, *et al.* Incidence of dementia and probable Alzheimer's disease in a general population: the Framingham study. *Neurology* 1993;43:515–19

25. Henderson VW, Paganini-Hill A, Emanuel CK, Dunn ME, Buckwalter JG. Estrogen replacement therapy in older women: comparisons between Alzheimer's disease cases and nondemented control subjects. *Arch Neurol* 1994;51:896–900

26. Ripich DN, Petrill SA, Whitehouse PJ, Ziol EW. Gender differences in language of AD patients: a longitudinal study. *Neurology* 1995;45:299–302

27. Henderson VW, Buckwalter JG. Cognitive deficits of men and women with Alzheimer's disease. *Neurology* 1994;44:90–6

28. Henderson VW, Sobel E, Buckwalter JG. Survival in Alzheimer's disease: longer for women than for men [abstr.]. *Ann Neurol* 1994;36:310

29. Henderson VW. Estrogen, cognition, and a woman's risk of Alzheimer's disease. *Am J Med* 1997;103(Suppl 3A):11–18

30. Toran-Allerand CD, Miranda RC, Bentham WDL, *et al.* Estrogen receptors colocalize with low-affinity nerve growth factor receptors in cholinergic neurons of the basal forebrain. *Proc Natl Acad Sci USA* 1992;89:4668–72

31. Sar M, Stumpf WE. Central noradrenergic neurones concentrate ^{3}H-oestradiol. *Nature (London)* 1981;289:500–2

32. Fink G, Sumner BEH, Rosie R, Grace O, Quinn JP. Estrogen control of central neurotransmission: effect on mood, mental state, and memory. *Cell Mol Neurobiol* 1996;16: 325–43

33. Bartus RT, Dean RL, Beer B, Lippa AD. The cholinergic hypothesis of geriatric memory dysfunction. *Science* 1981;217:208–17

34. Coyle JT, Price DL, DeLong MR. Alzheimer's disease: a disorder of cortical cholinergic innervation. *Science* 1983;219:1184–90

35. Luine V. Estradiol increases choline acetyltransferase activity in specific basal forebrain nuclei and projection areas of female rats. *Exp Neurol* 1985;89:484–90

36. Gibbs RB, Pfaff DW. Effects of estrogen and fimbria/fornix transection on p75[NGFR] and ChAT expression in the medial septum and diagonal band of Broca. *Exp Neurol* 1992; 116:23–39

37. Gibbs RB, Hashash A, Johnson DA. Effects of estrogen on potassium-stimulated acetylcholine release in the hippocampus and overlying cortex of adult rats. *Brain Res* 1996;749: 143–6

38. Singh M, Meyer EM, Millard WJ, Simpkins JW. Ovarian steroid deprivation results in a reversible learning impairment and compromised cholinergic function in female Sprague–Dawley rats. *Brain Res* 1994;644:305–12

39. Garcia-Segura LM, Cardona-Gomez P, Naftolin F, Chowen JA. Estradiol upregulates Bcl-2 expression in adult brain neurons. *NeuroReport* 1998;9:593–7

40. Tuszynski MH, U HS, Yoshida K, Gage FH. Recombinant human nerve growth factor infusions prevent cholinergic neuronal degeneration in the adult primate brain. *Ann Neurol* 1991;30:625–36

41. Knusel B, Beck KD, Winslow JW, et al. Brain-derived neurotrophic factor administration protects basal forebrain cholinergic but not nigral dopaminergic neurons from degenerative changes after axotomy in the adult rat brain. *J Neurosci* 1992;12:4391–402

42. Olson L, Nordberg A, von Holst H, et al. Nerve growth factor affects 11C-nicotine binding, blood flow, EEG and verbal episodic memory in an Alzheimer patient. *J Neural Trans* 1992;4:79–95

43. Miranda RC, Sohrabji F, Toran-Allerand CD. Presumptive estrogen target neurons express mRNAs for both the neurotrophins and neurotrophin receptors: a basis for potential developmental interactions of estrogen with neurotrophins. *Mol Cell Neurosci* 1993;4:510–25

44. Salehi A, Verhaagen J, Dijkhuizen PA, Swaab DF. Co-localization of high-affinity neurotrophin receptors in nucleus basalis of Meynert neurons and their differential reduction in Alzheimer's disease. *Neuroscience* 1996;75:373–87

45. McMillan PJ, Singer CA, Dorsa DM. The effects of ovariectomy and estrogen replacement on trkA and choline acetyltransferase mRNA expression in the basal forebrain of the adult female Sprague–Dawley rat. *J Neurosci* 1996;16:1860–5

46. Ferreira A, Caceres A. Estrogen-enhanced neurite growth: evidence for a selective induction of tau and stable microtubules. *J Neurosci* 1991;11:393–400

47. Xu H, Gouras GK, Greenfield JP, et al. Estrogen reduces neuronal generation of Alzheimer β-amyloid peptides. *Nature Med* 1998;4:447–51

48. Muesing RA, Miller VT, LaRosa JC, Stoy DB, Phillips EA. Effects of unopposed conjugated equine estrogen on lipoprotein composition and apolipoprotein-E distribution. *J Clin Endocrinol Metab* 1992;75:1250–4

49. Stone DJ, Rozovsky I, Morgan TE, Anderson CP, Hajian H, Finch CE. Astrocytes and microglia respond to estrogen with increased apoE mRNA *in vivo* and *in vitro*. *Exp Neurol* 1997;143:313–18

50. Poirier J, Hess M, May PC, Finch CE. Astrocytic apolipoprotein E mRNA and GFAP mRNA in hippocampus after entorhinal cortex lesioning. *Mol Brain Res* 1991;11:97–106

51. Stone DJ, Rozovsky I, Morgan TE, Anderson CP, Finch CE. Increased synaptic sprouting in response to estrogen via an apolipoprotein E dependent mechanism: implications for Alzheimer's disease. *J Neurosci* 1998;18:3180–5

52. Blennow K, Hesse C, Fredman P. Cerebrospinal fluid apolipoprotein E is reduced in Alzheimer's disease. *NeuroReport* 1994;5:2534–6

53. Bertrand P, Poirier J, Oda T, Finch CE, Pasinetti GM. Association of apolipoprotein E genotype with brain levels of apolipoprotein E and apolipoprotein J (clusterin) in Alzheimer disease. *Mol Brain Res* 1995;33:174–8

54. Bauer J, Ganter U, Strauss S, *et al.* The participation of interleukin-6 in the pathogenesis of Alzheimer's disease. *Res Immunol* 1992;143:650–7

55. Josefsson E, Tarkowski A, Carlsten H. Anti-inflammatory properties of estrogen. *Cell Immunol* 1992;142:67–78

56. Gilmore W, Weiner LP, Correale J. Effect of estradiol on cytokine secretion by proteolipid protein-specific T cell clones isolated from multiple sclerosis patients and normal control subjects. *J Immunol* 1997;158:446–51

57. Smith MA, Harris PLR, Sayre LM, Beckman JS, Perry G. Widespread peroxynitrite-mediated damage in Alzheimer's disease. *J Neurosci* 1997;17:2653–7

58. McDonald DR, Brunden KR, Landreth GE. Amyloid fibrils activate tyrosine kinase-dependent signaling and superoxide production in microglia. *J Neurosci* 1997;17:2284–94

59. Sagara Y, Dargusch R, Klier FG, Schubert D, Behl C. Increased antioxidant enzyme activity in amyloid β protein-resistant cells. *J Neurosci* 1996;16:497–505

60. Niki E, Nakano M. Estrogens as antioxidants. *Method Enzymol* 1990;186:330–3

61. Mooradian AD. Antioxidant properties of steroids. *J Steroid Biochem Mol Biol* 1993;45:509–11

62. Sack MN, Rader DJ, Cannon ROI. Oestrogen and inhibition of oxidation of low-density lipoproteins in postmenopausal women. *Lancet* 1994;343:269–70

63. Lindheim SR, Legro RS, Bernstein L, *et al.* Behavioral stress responses in premenopausal and postmenopausal women and the effects of estrogen. *Am J Obstet Gynecol* 1992;167:1831–6

64. Davis KL, Davis BM, Greenwald BS, *et al.* Cortisol and Alzheimer's disease. I: Basal studies. *Am J Psychiatry* 1986;143:300–5

65. Heuser IJ, Litvan I, Juncos JL, *et al.* Cortisol baseline secretion and memory performance in patients with dementia of the Alzheimer type. In Agnoli A, Cahn J, Lassen N, Mayeux R, eds. *Senile Dementias: II International Symposium*. Paris: John Libbey Eurotext, 1988:351–3

66. de Leon MJ, McRae T, Tasi JR, *et al.* Abnormal cortisol response in Alzheimer's disease linked to hippocampal atrophy [Letter]. *Lancet* 1988;2:391–2

67. Lupien S, Lecours AR, Lussier I, Schwartz G, Nair NPV, Meaney MJ. Basal cortisol levels and cognitive deficits in human aging. *J Neurosci* 1994;14:2893–903

68. McEwen BS, Sapolsky RM. Stress and cognitive function. *Curr Opin Neurobiol* 1995;5:205–16

69. White L, Petrovitch H, Ross GW, Masaki K. Association of mid-life consumption of tofu with late life cognitive impairment and dementia: the Honolulu–Asia Study [abstr]. *Neurobiol Aging* 1996;17(Suppl):S121

70. Hemminki E, Malin M, Topo P. Selection to postmenopausal therapy by women's characteristics. *J Clin Epidemiol* 1993;46:211–19

71. Derby CA, Hume AL, McPhillips JB, Barbour MM, Carleton RA. Prior and current health characteristics of postmenopausal estrogen replacement therapy users compared with nonusers. *Am J Obstet Gynecol* 1995;173:544–50

72. Birge SJ. The role of estrogen deficiency in the aging central nervous system. In Lobo RA, ed. *Treatment of the Postmenopausal Woman: Basic and Clinical Aspects.* New York: Raven Press, 1994:153–7

73. Mortel KF, Meyer JS. Lack of postmenopausal estrogen replacement therapy and the risk of dementia. *J Neuropsychiatr Clin Neurosci* 1995;7:334–7

74. Lerner A, Koss E, Debanne S, Rowland D, Smyth K, Friedland R. Smoking and oestrogen-replacement therapy as protective factors for Alzheimer's disease [Letter]. *Lancet* 1997;349:403–4

75. Baldereschi M, Di Carlo A, Lepore V, et al. Estrogen-replacement therapy and Alzheimer's disease in the Italian Longitudinal Study on Aging. *Neurology* 1998;50: 996–1002

76. Paganini-Hill A, Henderson VW. Estrogen deficiency and risk of Alzheimer's disease in women. *Am J Epidemiol* 1994;140:256–61

77. Brenner DE, Kukull WA, Stergachis A, et al. Postmenopausal estrogen replacement therapy and the risk of Alzheimer's disease: a population-based case–control study. *Am J Epidemiol* 1994;140:262–7

78. Tang M-X, Jacobs D, Stern Y, et al. Effect of oestrogen during menopause on risk and age at onset of Alzheimer's disease. *Lancet* 1996;348:429–32

79. Paganini-Hill A, Henderson VW. Estrogen replacement therapy and risk of Alzheimer's disease. *Arch Intern Med* 1996;156:2213–17

80. Kawas C, Resnick S, Morrison A, et al. A prospective study of estrogen replacement therapy and the risk of developing Alzheimer's disease: the Baltimore Longitudinal Study of Aging. *Neurology* 1997;48:1517–21

81. Waring SC, Rocca WA, Petersen RC, Kokmen E. Postmenopausal estrogen replacement therapy and Alzheimer's disease: a population-based study in Rochester, Minnesota [abstr]. *Neurology* 1997;48(Suppl 2):A79

82. Henderson VW, Watt L, Buckwalter JG. Cognitive skills associated with estrogen replacement in women with Alzheimer's disease. *Psychoneuroendocrinology* 1996;21:421–30

83. Fillit H, Weinreb H, Cholst I, et al. Observations in a preliminary open trial of estradiol therapy for senile dementia – Alzheimer's type. *Psychoneuroendocrinology* 1986;11:337–45

84. Honjo H, Ogino Y, Naitoh K, et al. In vivo effects by estrone sulfate on the central nervous system – senile dementia (Alzheimer's type). *J Steroid Biochem* 1989;34:521–5

85. Honjo H, Ogino Y, Tanaka K, et al. An effect of conjugated estrogen to cognitive impairment in women with senile dementia – Alzheimer's type: a placebo-controlled double blind study. *J Jpn Menopause Soc* 1993;1:167–71

86. Ohkura T, Isse K, Akazawa K, Hamamoto M, Yaoi Y, Hagino N. Low-dose estrogen replacement therapy for Alzheimer disease in women. *Menopause* 1994;1:125–30

87. Ohkura T, Isse K, Akazawa K, Hamamoto M, Yaoi Y, Hagino N. Evaluation of estrogen treatment in female patients with dementia of the Alzheimer type. *Endocr J* 1994;41: 361–71

88. Ohkura T, Isse K, Akazawa K, Hamamoto M, Yaoi Y, Hagino N. Long-term estrogen replacement therapy in female patients with dementia of the Alzheimer type: 7 case reports. *Dementia* 1995;6:99–107

89. Henderson VW. Estrogen replacement therapy for the prevention and treatment of Alzheimer's disease. *CNS Drugs* 1997;8:343–51

90. Asthana S, Craft S, Baker LD, *et al.* Transdermal estrogen improves memory in women with Alzheimer's disease [abstr]. *Soc Neurosci Abstr* 1996;22:200

91. Birge SJ. The role of estrogen in the treatment of Alzheimer's disease. *Neurology* 1997; 48(Suppl 7):S36–41

92. Dohanich GP, Fader AJ, Javorsky DJ. Estrogen and estrogen–progesterone treatments counteract the effect of scopolamine on reinforced T-maze alternation in female rats. *Behav Neurosci* 1994;108:988–92

93. Fader AJ, Hendricson AW, Dohanich GP. Estrogen improves performance of reinforced T-maze alternation and prevents the amnestic effects of scopolamine administered systemically or intrahippocampally. *Neurobiol Learn Memory* 1998;69:225–40

94. Packard MG. Posttraining estrogen and memory modulation. *Horm Behav* 1998;34: 126–39

95. Knapp MJ, Knopman DS, Solomon PR, Pendlebury WW, Davis CS, Garcon SI. A 30-week randomized controlled trial of high-dose tacrine in patients with Alzheimer's disease. *J Am Med Assoc* 1994;271:985–91

96. Rogers SL, Farlow MR, Doody RS, Mohs R, Friedhoff LT, Group DS. A 24-week, double-blind, placebo-controlled trial of donepezil in patients with Alzheimer's disease. *Neurology* 1998;50:136–45

97. Schneider LS, Farlow MR, Henderson VW, Pogoda JM. Effects of estrogen replacement therapy on response to tacrine in patients with Alzheimer's disease. *Neurology* 1996;46: 1580–4

98. Ohkura T, Isse K, Akazawa K, Hamamoto M, Yaoi Y, Hagino N. An open trial of estrogen therapy for dementia of the Alzheimer type in women. In Berg G, Hammar M, eds. *The Modern Management of the Menopause: A Perspective for the 21st Century.* Carnforth, UK: Parthenon Publishing, 1994:315–33

99. Woolley CS, McEwen BS. Roles of estradiol and progesterone in regulation of hippocampal dendritic spine density during the estrous cycle in the rat. *J Comp Neurol* 1993; 336:293–306

100. Gibbs RB. Fluctuations in relative levels of choline acetyltransferase mRNA in different regions of the rat basal forebrain across the estrus cycle: effects of estrogen and progestrone. *J Neurosci* 1996;16:1049–55

101. Meldrum DR, Davidson BJ, Tataryn IV, Judd HL. Changes in circulating steroids with aging in postmenopausal women. *Obstet Gynecol* 1981;57:624–8

102. Kopelman PG, White N, Pilkington TRE, Jeffcoate SL. The effect of weight loss on sex steroid secretion and binding in massively obese women. *Clin Endocrinol* 1981;14:113–16

103. Berlinger WG, Potter JF. Low body mass index in demented outpatients. *J Am Geriatr Soc* 1991:973–8

104. Buckwalter JG, Schneider LS, Wilshire TW, Dunn ME, Henderson VW. Body weight, estrogen and cognitive functioning in Alzheimer's disease: an analysis of the tacrine study group. *Arch Gerontol Geriatr* 1997;24:261–7

105. van Duijn C, Meijer H, Witteman JCM, *et al.* Estrogen, apolipoprotein E and the risk of Alzheimer's disease [abstr]. *Neurobiol Aging* 1996;17(Suppl):S79–80

6
Cerebrovascular disease

Cerebrovascular disease, or stroke, is disease of the brain caused by pathological changes in the blood or blood vessels. The brain represents about 2.5% of body weight, receives 15% of the cardiac output and consumes 20% of the oxygen. Its high metabolic rate renders the brain critically dependent on the cerebral circulation to supply oxygen and glucose. Cessation of cerebral blood flow for as little as 5 min results in neuronal death. As discussed further below, several estrogen properties may influence the risk of stroke or be neuroprotective in the setting of acute stroke. Hormone effects on other forms of vascular disease (cardiovascular disease, systemic venous thrombosis) are also considered below in the context of stroke.

At age 50 years, a woman faces an estimated 20% probability of developing a stroke within her lifetime and an 8% probability of dying from a stroke[1]. The two major types of stroke are infarction and hemorrhage (Table 6.1). For infarction, ischemic injury occurs as a direct consequence of diminished blood flow. For hemorrhage, vascular rupture into the subarachnoid space or brain parenchyma causes neuronal death through tissue compression, secondary vasospasm and other mechanisms. Both infarction and hemorrhage are primarily diseases of the arterial system; venous stroke occurs infrequently. In Western countries, stroke is the third leading cause of death, exceeded only by ischemic heart disease and cancer.

Occlusion of a large intracranial artery by an embolus is a principal cause of cerebral infarction. Emboli commonly originate from the heart. Atrial fibrillation, valvular disease, or myocardial infarction are among various factors that predispose to the formation of cardiac thrombi, which subsequently dislodge as blood-borne emboli to the brain. An artery-to-artery embolus is another common cause of cerebral vascular occlusion, an event referred to as an atherothrombotic stroke. Composed of platelets, fibrin, atheromatous material, or thrombus, these emboli typically arise within extracranial portions of the carotid or vertebral artery from the ulcerated surface of an atheromatous plaque. Occlusion of a small intracranial artery (e.g. one of the lenticulostriate branches of the middle cerebral artery) is

Table 6.1. Causes of stroke

Common causes of stroke
Cerebral infarction
    Occlusion of a large artery
        embolic stroke: embolus from the heart or another systemic source
        atherothrombotic stroke: atherosclerosis within large extracranial vessels and
            subsequent artery-to-artery embolus
    Occlusion of a small artery
        lacunar stroke: usually atherosclerosis and fibrinoid necrosis of a small pene-
            trating artery
Cerebral hemorrhage
    Hemorrhage predominantly into the subarachnoid space
        berry aneurysm of large artery
        vascular malformation
    Hemorrhage predominantly within the brain parenchyma
        microaneurysm of small penetrating artery ('hypertensive' hemorrhage)

Uncommon causes of stroke
Venous sinus occlusion, hematological disorders, vasculitis, trauma, migraine,
    others

usually not due to an embolus but instead is associated with hypertension-induced atheroma or fibrinoid necrosis affecting the vascular wall directly.

Causes of cerebral hemorrhage include the rupture of a berry aneurysm, which has developed over time at the site of congenital defect in the vessel wall, the rupture of a vascular malformation, or the rupture of a small artery whose wall has been weakened by the presence of long-standing hypertension.

PREVENTION OF STROKE

Whether estrogen helps prevent stroke or actually increases the risk of stroke depends on a number of factors, including the woman's age and the type of stroke under consideration. From a population point of view, the potentially most important impact of estrogen would be after the menopause, when the incidence of stroke is greatest.

Estrogen influences various factors involved in the coagulation cascade and fibrinolysis[2–4]. The net effect of estrogen is to increase vascular risk among current users, particularly in the systemic venous system. Use of oral contraceptives increases the rate of deep vein thrombosis and pulmonary embolism[5]. Oral contraceptives also elevate the younger woman's risk of ischemic stroke[6,7]. Fortunately, the incidence of life-threatening thromboembolism is quite low, even among pill-users. Not all estrogens are alike, and oral contraceptives may be more potent contributors to vascular risk than popular preparations of hormone replacement therapy used by older women[8]. Nevertheless, after the menopause estrogen therapy also increases the risk of systemic venous thrombosis, but as in younger women the actual incidence is low[9–12]. The impact of estrogen on stroke risk in older women is considered below.

During pregnancy, the incidence of ischemic stroke does not change, while that of intracerebral hemorrhage may be somewhat elevated[13,14]. Pregnancy is also associated with a heightened risk of subarachnoid hemorrhage from a vascular malformation[15]. In the postpartum period, however, the risk of both ischemic and hemorrhagic stroke is elevated[14]. Most infarcts are due to arterial rather than to venous occlusion[16]. During pregnancy and after delivery, eclampsia is an important risk factor for stroke. Other factors that contribute to stroke risk include changes in the vascular wall[17], altered levels of clotting factors and fibrinogen, and hemodynamic changes.

Stroke prevention after the menopause

The incidence of stroke climbs steeply with age[18] (Figure 6.1). Rates are lower for women than men, although after the menopause rates tend to converge. Hypertension, a particularly important risk factor for stroke, increases the risk of cerebral infarction primarily by accelerating the development of atheroma near vascular curves and branch points, where blood flow is turbulent and shearing forces are increased. The site where the common carotid artery bifurcates into internal and external branches is especially vulnerable to atherothrombotic changes.

Convincing observational data testify to the substantial importance of post-menopausal estrogen therapy for the primary prevention of cardiovascular disease[19]. Because coronary artery disease and cerebrovascular disease share common risk factors, it might be expected that estrogen should be equally protective against stroke. However, shared risk factors for cardiovascular and cerebrovascular disease

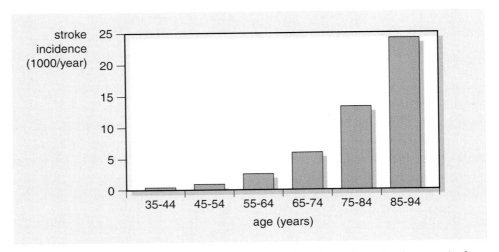

Figure 6.1. Incidence of stroke in women as a function of age in the Framingham study. Data are from reference 18

are primarily those linked to atherosclerosis, and data supporting a role for estrogen in stroke prevention are less compelling than for cardiovascular disease.

Extrapolating largely from laboratory and clinical studies on vascular disease and vascular function, estrogens might modify the risk of cerebral infarction through competing effects on coagulation and fibrinolysis[2–4]. Theoretically, estrogen effects on lipids and the vascular wall should reduce stroke risk through reduction of atherosclerotic disease and augmentation of cerebral blood flow (Table 6.2). Estrogen reduces levels of low-density lipoprotein (LDL)–cholesterol and increases levels of high-density lipoprotein (HDL)–cholesterol[2]. Both actions favorably impact on atherosclerosis. Estrogen also lowers serum levels of lipoprotein(a)[2], another important cardiovascular risk factor. Congruent with these laboratory findings, clinical observations confirm that estrogen therapy significantly reduces atherosclerotic narrowing of the coronary[20] and carotid[21–23] arteries (Figure 6.2).

When cardioprotective effects of hormone replacement therapy after the menopause are considered, benefit substantially exceeds that predicted on the basis of alterations of the lipid profile[24]. Estrogen effects on coronary artery smooth muscle may be of paramount importance in cardioprotection. At physiological concentrations, estrogen leads to arterial vasodilatation through mechanisms both dependent upon, and independent of, the vascular endothelium. One key action is to enhance the availability of nitric oxide, an endothelium-derived relaxing

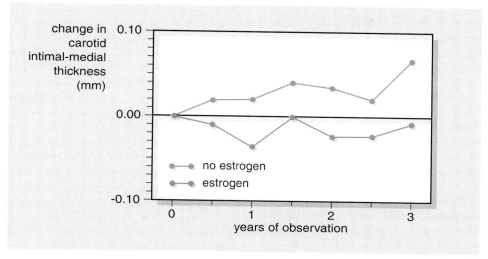

Figure 6.2. Estrogen replacement and change in intimal–medial thickness of the carotid artery. Change in the width of the carotid intima–media is thought to reflect underlying atherosclerosis. Mean changes from baseline were determined by ultrasonography. Unlike estrogen users, women who reported no estrogen use showed increased intimal–medial thickness over the 3-year period of observation. Redrawn from reference 22

factor[25]. In the coronary arteries, the net effect is increased blood flow and reduced likelihood of vasoconstriction and thrombus formation. Similar effects presumably occur in the intracranial circulation. Furthermore, estrogen has other, long-term, effects on the arterial wall. As imaged by high-resolution ultrasonography of the carotid artery[26], hormone replacement is associated with thinning of the intima layer, as well as with thickening of the media, a layer characterized by its smooth muscle, collagen and elastin content. The media plays a nutritive role for the intima, and estrogen effects on these two layers may help retard atherosclerotic buildup.

What are the actual effects of postmenopausal estrogen therapy on stroke risk? Epidemiological studies suggest that fatal stroke among estrogen users is reduced by 20–60%[27]. The protective impact of estrogen on stroke mortality is evident across studies. However, estrogen effects on stroke incidence (as opposed to mortality) are inconsistent, and indeed several major studies failed to confirm a significant benefit[27].

In part, discrepancies between cardioprevention and neuroprevention reflect a failure or inability to distinguish among various causes of stroke. However, even for ischemic disease, mechanisms and risk factors differ between heart and brain[28], and, interestingly, gender differences in the risk of ischemic brain disease are much less pronounced than differences in the rate of ischemic heart disease[18] (Figure 6.3). Coronary occlusion leading to myocardial infarction is most often due to ulceration of an atherosclerotic plaque followed by acute thrombosis[29]. Although a similar process often occurs in cerebral infarction, only a subset of ischemic strokes are actually due to atherothrombosis[30]. Thus, even well-designed epidemiological studies limited to cerebral infarction have failed to discern the degree of risk reduction anticipated on the basis of studies of ischemic heart disease. In the Nurses' Health Study, women using estrogen replacement experienced a risk of coronary artery disease that was significantly (40%) lower than non-users' risk, whereas the risk of ischemic stroke in this large cohort was not at all reduced among current or past estrogen users[31]. Similarly, a case–control study from the Kaiser Permanente health-care group reported that neither current estrogen use nor prior use significantly influenced the risk of ischemic stroke[32].

Stroke prevention in men

Interestingly, estrogens at one time were considered for use in men, based on favorable estrogenic effects on atherosclerosis. A secondary prevention trial involved 582 men with recent cerebral infarction[33]. In this randomized study,

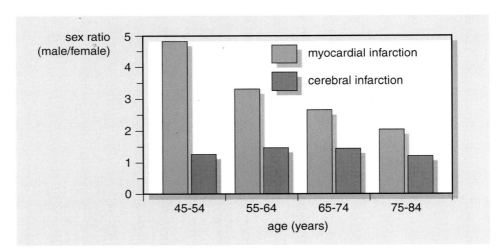

Figure 6.3. Sex differences in the incidence of myocardial and cerebral infarction as a function of age. In the Framingham study, there was a striking male preponderance for myocardial infarction, but for atherothrombotic stroke, the male-to-female sex ratio was less elevated. Data are from reference 18

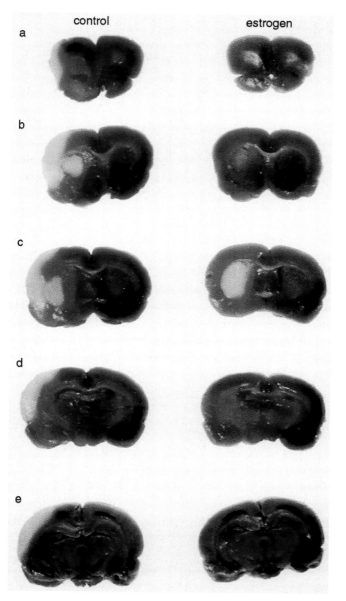

control estrogen

a

b

c

d

e

Figure 6.4. Effect of estrogen on experimental cerebral infarction. Ovariectomized rats were injected with estradiol or vehicle before unilateral occlusion of the middle cerebral artery; 24 h later, the animals were sacrificed. In coronal sections of the brain (**a–e**), ischemic regions (white) failed to take up the 2,3,5-triphenyl tetrazolium chloride stain. Viable brain areas stained red. Representative sections from a vehicle-treated animal are displayed on the left, and those of an animal treated with estradiol on the right. Cortical infarct size is reduced in the animal that received estrogen. Reproduced with permission from reference 38

patients received conjugated estrogens (1.25–2.5 mg/day) or placebo. Over an average follow-up period of 17 months, however, there was no significant positive or negative effect of active treatment on recurrent stroke or on other defined endpoints.

NEUROPROTECTION AFTER STROKE

There is mounting evidence that estrogen can protect the ischemic brain. Cerebral infarction is less extensive in female animals than in males[34–36]. In experimental models, ovariectomy increased infarct size[36], whereas estrogen administered to ovariectomized animals prior to or immediately after vascular occlusion significantly reduced both infarct size and stroke mortality[37] (Figure 6.4).

Several estrogen actions may help preserve neuronal function in the setting of acute ischemia (Table 6.2). Neuroprotection depends on preserving damaged but potentially viable neurons. Estrogen increases the active transport of glucose into the brain[38] and boosts cerebral blood flow[39–42]. In experimental cerebral ischemia, supraphysiological levels of estrogen augment blood flow initially and reduce the degree of subsequent hyperemic reperfusion[43]. Other neuroprotective effects may depend on the ability of estrogen to reduce free radical damage[44–47] and to ameliorate toxicity mediated by excitatory neurotransmitters[47].

Although animal models have focused on ischemic stroke, some estrogen properties could also be protective in the setting of cerebral hemorrhage, where vasospasm and tissue compression by an intracranial clot secondarily interfere with cerebral perfusion.

Table 6.2. Estrogen actions that may influence stroke risk and outcome

---

Stroke prevention
Competing effects on coagulation and fibrinolysis
More favorable lipid profile
Short- and long-term effects on vascular wall

Stroke outcome
Increased cerebral blood flow
Increased glucose transport into the brain
Antioxidant effects
Reduced excitotoxicity

REFERENCES

1. Grady D, Rubin SM, Petitti DB, *et al.* Hormone therapy to prevent disease and prolong life in postmenopausal women. *Ann Intern Med* 1992;117:1016–37
2. Nabulsi AA, Folsom AR, White A, *et al.* Association of hormone-replacement therapy with various cardiovascular risk factors in postmenopausal women. *N Engl J Med* 1993;328: 1069–75
3. Lindoff C, Peterson F, Lecander I, Martinsson G, Astedt B. Transdermal estrogen replacement therapy: beneficial effects on hemostatic risk factors for cardiovascular disease. *Maturitas* 1996;24:43–50
4. Koh KK, Mincemoyer R, Bui MN, *et al.* Effects of hormone-replacement therapy on fibrinolysis in postmenopausal women. *N Engl J Med* 1997;336:683–90
5. World Health Organization Collaborative Study. Venous thromboembolic disease and combined oral contraceptives: results of international multicentre case–control study. *Lancet* 1995;346:1575–82
6. Collaborative Group for the Study of Stroke in Young Women. Oral contraception and increased risk of cerebral ischemia or thrombosis. *N Engl J Med* 1973;288:871–8
7. Lidegaard O. Oral contraception and risk of a cerebral thromboembolic attack: results of a case–control study. *Br Med J* 1993;306:956–63
8. Lobo RA. Estrogen and the risk of coagulopathy. *Am J Med* 1992;92:283–6
9. Daly E, Vessey MP, Hawkins MM, Carson JL, Gough P, Marsh S. Risk of venous thromboembolism in users of hormone replacement therapy. *Lancet* 1996;348:977–80
10. Grodstein F, Stampfer MJ, Goldhaber SZ, *et al.* Prospective study of exogenous hormones and risk of pulmonary embolism in women. *Lancet* 1996;348:983–7
11. Jick H, Derbey LE, Myers MW, Vasilakis C, Newton KM. Risk of hospital admission for idiopathic venous thromboembolism among users of postmenopausal oestrogens. *Lancet* 1996;348:981–3
12. Pérez Gutthann S, Rodríguez LAG, Castellsague J, Oliart AD. Hormone replacement therapy and risk of venous thromboembolism: population based case–control study. *Br Med J* 1996;314:796–800
13. Sharshar T, Lamy C, Mas JL. Incidence and causes of strokes associated with pregnancy and puerperium: a study in public hospitals of Ile de France. *Stroke* 1995;26:930–6
14. Kittner SJ, Stern BJ, Feeser BR, *et al.* Pregnancy and the risk of stroke. *N Engl J Med* 1996; 335:768–74
15. Robinson JL, Hall CS, Sedzimir CB. Arteriovenous malformations, aneurysms, and pregnancy. *J Neurosurg* 1974;41:63–70
16. Cross JN, Castro PO, Jennett WB. Cerebral strokes associated with pregnancy and the puerperium. *Br Med J* 1968;3:214–18
17. Irey NS, Norris HJ. Intimal vascular lesions associated with female reproductive steroids. *Arch Pathol* 1973;96:227–34
18. Wolf PA, D'Agostino RB. Epidemiology of stroke. In Barnett HJM, Mohr JP, Stein BM, Yatsu FM, eds. *Stroke: Pathophysiology, Diagnosis, and Management.* New York: Churchill Livingstone, 1998:3–28
19. Grodstein F, Stampfer M. The epidemiology of coronary heart disease and estrogen replacement in postmenopausal women. *Prog Cardiovasc Dis* 1995;38:199–210

20. Sullivan JM. Coronary arteriography in estrogen-treated postmenopausal women. *Prog Cardiovasc Dis* 1995;38:211–22

21. Manolio TA, Furberg CD, Shemanski L, *et al.* Associations of postmenopausal estrogen use with cardiovascular disease and its risk factors in older women. *Circulation* 1993;88:2163–71

22. Espeland MA, Applegate W, Furberg CD, Lefkowitz D, Rice L, Hunninghake D. Estrogen replacement therapy and progression of intimal–medial thickness in the carotid arteries of postmenopausal women. *Am J Epidemiol* 1995;142:1011–19

23. Akkad A, Hartshorne T, Bell PRF, Al-Azzawi F. Carotid plaque regression on oestrogen replacement: a pilot study. *Eur J Vasc Endovasc Surg* 1996;13:347–8

24. Bush TL, Barrett-Conner E, Cowan LD, *et al.* Cardiovascular mortality and noncontraceptive use of estrogen in women: results from the Lipid Research Clinics Program Follow-up Study. *Circulation* 1987;75:1102–9

25. Guetta V, Quyyumi AA, Prasad A, Panza JA, Waclawiw M, Cannon RO III. The role of nitric oxide in coronary vascular effects of estrogen in postmenopausal women. *Circulation* 1997;96:2795–801

26. Baron YM, Galea R, Brincat M. Carotid artery wall changes in estrogen treated and untreated postmenopausal women. *Obstet Gynecol* 1998;91:982–6

27. Paganini-Hill A. Estrogen replacement therapy and stroke. *Prog Cardiovasc Dis* 1995;38:223–42

28. Puddu P, Puddu GM, Bastagli L, Massarelli G, Muscari A. Coronary and cerebrovascular atherosclerosis: two aspects of the same disease or two different pathologies? *Arch Gerontol Geriatr* 1995;20:15–22

29. Falk E. Plaque rupture with severe pre-existing stenosis precipitating coronary thrombosis: characteristics of coronary atherosclerotic plaques underlying fatal occlusive thrombi. *Br Heart J* 1983;50:127–34

30. Adams RD, Victor M, Ropper AH. *Principles of Neurology*, 6th edn. New York: McGraw-Hill, 1997

31. Grodstein F, Stampfer MJ, Manson JE, *et al.* Postmenopausal estrogen and progestin use and the risk of cardiovascular disease. *N Engl J Med* 1996;335:453–61

32. Petitti DB, Sidney S, Quesenberry CPJ, Bernstein A. Ischemic stroke and use of estrogen and estrogen/progestogen as hormone replacement therapy. *Stroke* 1998;29:23–8

33. Veterans Administration Cooperative Study of Atherosclerosis – Neurology Section. An evaluation of estrogenic substances in the treatment of cerebral vascular disease. *Circulation* 1966;33(Suppl 2):3–9

34. Hall ED, Pazara KE, Linseman KL. Sex differences in postischemic neuronal necrosis in gerbils. *J Cereb Blood Flow Metab* 1991;11:292–8

35. Li K, Futrell N, Tovar JS, Wang LC, Wang DZ, Schultz LR. Gender influences the magnitude of the inflammatory response within embolic infarcts in young rats. *Stroke* 1996;27:498–503

36. Alkayed NJ, Harukuni I, Kimes AS, London ED, Traystman RJ, Hurn PD. Gender-linked brain injury in experimental stroke. *Stroke* 1998;29:159–66

37. Simpkins JW, Rajakumar G, Zhang Y-Q, *et al.* Estrogens may reduce mortality and ischemic damage caused by middle cerebral artery occlusion in the female rat. *J Neurosurg* 1997;87:724–30

38. Shi J, Simpkins JW. 17β-Estradiol modulation of glucose transporter 1 expression in blood–brain barrier. *Am J Physiol* 1997;272:E1016–22

39. Belfort MA, Saade GR, Snabes M, *et al.* Hormonal status affects the reactivity of the cerebral vasculature. *Am J Obstet Gynecol* 1995;172:1273–8

40. Ohkura T, Isse K, Akazawa K, Hamamoto M, Yaoi Y, Hagino N. Evaluation of estrogen treatment in female patients with dementia of the Alzheimer type. *Endocr J* 1994;41:361–71

41. Ohkura T, Teshima Y, Isse K, *et al.* Estrogen increases cerebral and cerebellar blood flows in postmenopausal women. *Menopause* 1995;2:13–18

42. Shamma FN, Fayad P, Brass L, Sarrel P. Middle cerebral artery blood velocity during controlled ovarian hyperstimulation. *Fertil Steril* 1992;57:1022–5

43. Hurn PD, Littleton-Kearney MT, Kirsch JR, Dharmarajan AM, Traystman RJ. Postischemic cerebral blood flow recovery in the female: effect of 17β-estradiol. *J Cereb Blood Flow Metab* 1995;15:666–72

44. Mukai K, Daifuku K, Yokoyama S, Nakano M. Stopped-flow investigation of antioxidant activity of estrogens in solution. *Biochim Biophys Acta* 1990;1035:348–52

45. Niki E, Nakano M. Estrogens as antioxidants. *Method Enzymol* 1990;186:330–3

46. Mooradian AD. Antioxidant properties of steroids. *J Steroid Biochem Mol Biol* 1993;45:509–11

47. Goodman Y, Bruce AJ, Cheng B, Mattson MP. Estrogens attenuate and corticosterone exacerbates excitotoxicity, oxidative injury, and amyloid β-peptide toxicity in hippocampal neurons. *J Neurochem* 1996;66:1836–44

7
Other neurological disorders

MOVEMENT DISORDERS

Motor and somatosensory systems of the brain work together to control body movements. Direct motor control is achieved through the corticospinal (and analogous corticobulbar) system, whose fibers originate from the cortex of the frontal and parietal lobes and descend through the medullary pyramids to synapse on motor neurons of the spinal cord. Corticospinal and corticobulbar input to lower-motor neurons is modulated at different levels. Particularly important is the extrapyramidal system, a set of subcortical nuclei and interconnecting pathways. The extrapyramidal system includes large neurons of the substantia nigra that release the neurotransmitter dopamine in projection sites of the striatum. The substantia nigra itself contains few estrogen receptors[1]. Nevertheless, there is strong evidence that estrogen modifies dopamine receptors, the activity of dopamine-containing neurons and motor behaviors mediated by dopamine[2–5].

Clinicians have long suspected an association between ovarian hormones and hyperkinetic movement disorders. Chorea gravidarum, with characteristic involuntary rhythmic movements of the limbs, appears during pregnancy and resolves during the puerperium[6,7]. Reversible chorea, which clinically resembles chorea gravidarum, is also reported with oral contraceptive use[8].

A much more common and important extrapyramidal illness is Parkinson's disease, a hypokinetic neurodegenerative disorder of the basal ganglia characterized by tremor of the resting limbs, rigidity, diminished voluntary movements and impaired postural reflexes. Biochemical abnormalities involve deficiencies of catecholamine neurotransmitters, and most parkinsonian symptoms are attributed to the prominent loss of dopamine-containing neurons of the substantia nigra. Drugs that increase dopamine reduce symptoms of Parkinson's disease. In contrast, chorea and certain other hyperkinetic movement disorders are typically exacerbated by dopaminergic drugs; these movement disorders may benefit from treatment with neuroleptic medications or other dopamine antagonists.

Although estrogen clearly modulates dopaminergic activity within the nigrostriatal system, evidence is weak that estrogen modifies symptoms of patients with movement disorders. Younger women with Parkinson's disease sometimes complain of increased symptoms preceding or concurrent with menstruation[9]. Case reports of women receiving neuroleptic drugs imply that parkinsonian symptoms may be precipitated by estrogen therapy[10] and that estrogen might aggravate symptoms of Parkinson's disease[11,12].

Estrogen may have some limited efficacy for the treatment of hyperkinetic dyskinesias. An open-label study of 20 men with tardive dyskinesia, a hyperkinetic disorder induced by chronic neuroleptic therapy, found a significant reduction in dyskinesias after 6 weeks of treatment with oral conjugated estrogens[13]. A second study of conjugated estrogens failed to show significant change among patients with hyperkinesias of diverse etiologies[12]. However, it was observed *post hoc* that estrogen treatment noticeably decreased dyskinesia scores in two of ten Huntington's disease patients and four of ten patients with tardive dyskinesia. Eight dystonic patients in the same study evinced no effect of therapy[12].

Experimentally, estradiol has been shown to protect against the loss of dopamine neurons induced by neurotoxins[14]. However, estrogen use after the menopause does not appear to affect the risk of uncomplicated Parkinson's disease. A community-based case–control study that compared cognitively intact women with idiopathic Parkinson's disease to healthy women found no association with estrogen replacement therapy[15]. However, when analyses were extended to include women who developed dementia after the onset of Parkinson's disease, estrogen appeared to protect against dementia. Parkinsonian symptoms are commonly observed in Alzheimer's patients, and demented patients with pathological features of Parkinson's disease often have concomitant neuropathological changes of Alzheimer's disease[16,17]. Although dementia in Parkinson's disease can be variously determined, one interpretation of findings in this study is that the favorable effects of estrogen on parkinsonian dementia were due to putative protective effects on co-existing Alzheimer's pathology (see Chapter 5).

EPILEPSY

Epilepsy is a chronic neurological disease characterized by recurrent seizures. A seizure represents an abrupt change in brain function caused by the disorderly discharge of cerebral neurons. During a seizure, the abnormal epileptic discharge results in involuntary muscle contractions, loss of consciousness, or other neurological symptoms.

Estrogens may deleteriously influence epilepsy. In animal studies, the intravenous administration of estrogen or the topical application of estrogen to the exposed surface of the cerebral cortex induced abnormal electrical discharges[18]. Estrogen lowers the seizure threshold[19] and potentiates the experimental induction of seizures[20,21]. In female rats, the ease with which seizures are induced by electrical stimulation of the cerebral cortex varies during the estrous cycle; seizures are most easily elicited (i.e. the threshold is lowest) during proestrus[22], when estradiol levels are at their peak.

Estrogen increases the excitability of hippocampal neurons[23,24]. Synaptic plasticity, as measured by long-term potentiation, is increased in female rats during proestrus[25]. Spiny protuberances located on dendrites are sites of excitatory synapses in the central nervous system. For pyramidal neurons of the CA1 region of the hippocampus, the number of spines on apical dendrites varies during the rat estrous cycle, with the peak spine density occurring during proestrus[26]. *In vivo* experiments confirm that spine density changes occur in response to estrogen[27].

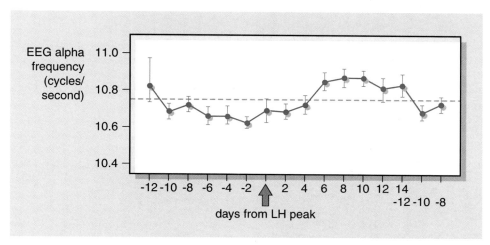

Figure 7.1. Effects of the menstrual cycle on background electroencephalographic (EEG) rhythms. The weighted mean alpha frequency (cycles/s), shown for 16 spontaneously cycling women, varies during the menstrual cycle. It is greatest during the luteal phase of the menstrual cycle. The arrow indicates the peak luteinizing hormone (LH) surge occurring immediately prior to ovulation, the dashed line indicates the mean frequency and error bars represent the standard error of the mean. Redrawn from reference 29

Based on laboratory findings such as these, estrogen is postulated to predispose to epilepsy by lowering the seizure threshold. Epilepsy often first develops at about the time of menarche[28]. Although slight changes in electroencephalographic rhythms can be detected during the menstrual cycle[29] (Figure 7.1), most epileptic women show no relationship between menstruation and seizures[30]. However, in the subset of patients with so-called catamenial epilepsy, seizure recurrence is closely linked to the menstrual cycle, being most likely to appear immediately preceding or during menstruation[28,31] (Figure 7.2). Catamenial seizures are thought to be triggered primarily by fluctuations in the concentrations of ovarian hormones[31,32]. In one study, intravenous estrogens were administered to a group of epileptic patients. Within seconds to minutes after injection, 11 of 16 patients developed epileptiform discharges on their electroencephalographic records[28]. In some patients, catamenial seizures may be unrelated to hormonal effects on the central nervous system. Rather, menstruation-associated fluctuations in serum concentrations of anticonvulsant medications could contribute to epileptic symptoms[33].

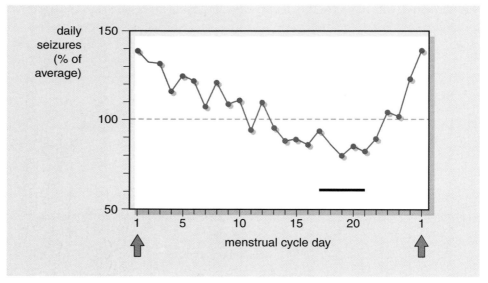

Figure 7.2. Frequency of seizures during different days of the menstrual cycle. In this study of 50 epileptic women, a total of 33 468 seizures were recorded over 9293 menstrual cycles. In the figure, the number of seizures on different days of the menstrual cycle is expressed as the percentage of the average number of daily seizures. Day 1 represents the first day of menstruation (arrow). The mid-luteal phase is indicated by the horizontal bar. Analyses were confined to 25 days surrounding the first day of menstruation. Redrawn from reference 31

Pregnancy is a time of heightened vulnerability to epilepsy[34] (Figure 7.3). Particularly among women whose epilepsy is poorly controlled before they become pregnant, seizure frequency commonly increases during this time[35]. A number of different explanations are offered for this exacerbation, including hormonal effects on the seizure threshold. However, other factors also increase the likelihood of seizures. Uncommonly, hormonally responsive neurological illnesses, such as cerebral thrombosis or the growth of a pre-existing meningioma (a hormonally responsive intracranial tumor) can be responsible. Other pregnancy-associated conditions that lead to seizures include sleep deprivation, eclampsia and declining serum concentrations of anticonvulsant medications.

In the laboratory, estrogen effects on epileptogenesis are opposed by progesterone[19,36]. Human observational studies[31,32] and preliminary treatment trials[37,38] also suggest that progestogens can reduce seizure frequency in epileptic women. In ovulating women, the ratio between estrogen and progesterone may also be important in determining seizure frequency, with a higher ratio associated with more seizures[32] (Figure 7.4).

The use of oral contraceptives by women with epilepsy does not increase the risk of seizures[39]. The effect of menopause on seizure frequency has not been well studied. However, menopause is not known to affect epilepsy symptoms to any substantial extent.

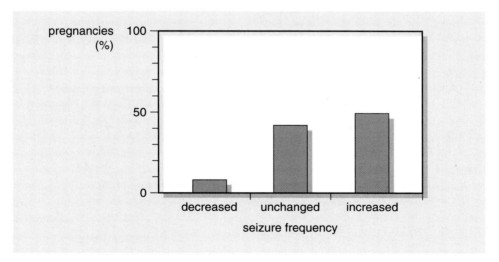

Figure 7.3. Effect of pregnancy on seizure frequency in women with pre-existing epilepsy. Percentages are based on 298 pregnancies reported in five clinical series, as summarized in reference 34

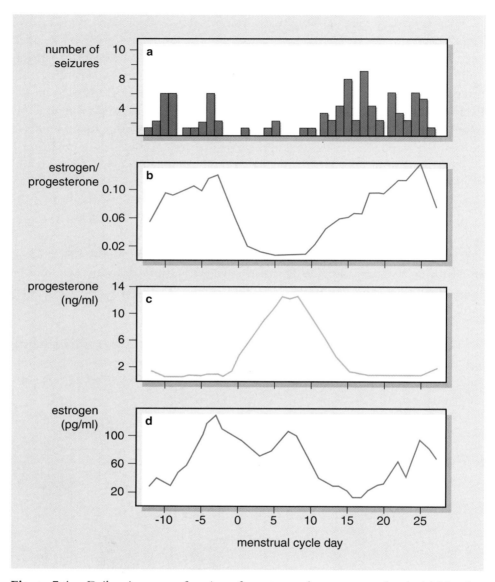

Figure 7.4. Daily seizures as a function of estrogen and progesterone levels. (**a**) Number of generalized seizures for six epileptic women on different days of the menstrual cycle. (**b**) Mean ratio of plasma estrogen to progesterone. (**c**) Progesterone levels. (**d**) Estrogen levels. On the x-axis, 0 represents the first cycle day that progesterone levels exceeded 2 ng/ml. Redrawn from reference 32

MIGRAINE HEADACHE

Migraine is characterized by recurrent throbbing head pain, often accompanied by gastrointestinal disturbances such as nausea, vomiting, or diarrhea. The term 'classic' migraine is used when unilateral pain is preceded by scintillating visual field defects or other focal neurological symptoms. When present, symptoms of the neurological aura tend to occur contralaterally to the ensuing head pain and last about 20 min. More commonly, pain is bilateral and not preceded by neurological disturbances.

Migraine pain is pulsatile in nature, and vascular factors are strongly implicated in headache pathogenesis. One common view is that the neurological aura reflects a period of intense vasoconstriction of intracranial vessels and that ensuing throbbing pain is due to distention and high-amplitude pulsation of the external carotid artery. Indeed, regional cerebral blood flow is consistently reduced during the aura of classic migraine. However, the pattern of blood flow during the ensuing headache phase is more variable, and regional flow does not necessarily increase at the onset of pain[40,41]. An alternative view is that the primary event of classic migraine is a focal depression of electrical activity. The area of electrical depression spreads slowly through the cerebral cortex, accompanied by regional reductions in cerebral blood flow[40,42]. Over-activity of the neurotransmitter serotonin is also implicated in migraine pathogenesis.

The prevalence of migraine is three times higher in women than men[43], and migraines appear to be hormonally influenced. Headache frequency is influenced by the menstrual cycle, pregnancy and the use of ovarian hormones. Estrogens have the potential to affect migraine headache through actions on cerebral blood flow[44,45] or on serotonergic activity[46–48].

For some women, migraine attacks appear to be triggered by estrogen withdrawal and are therefore especially apt to occur immediately before or during the menses[49–51] (Figure 7.5). Declining levels of progesterone may also play a role[52]. Treatment with estrogen can sometimes postpone or prevent attacks of premenstrual and menstrual migraine[53,54] (Figure 7.6). In one case report, sublingual estradiol aborted migraine symptoms in parallel with increases in middle cerebral artery flow, as documented by transcranial Doppler ultrasound measurements[55]. Perhaps owing to fluctuating estrogen levels, migraine frequency may worsen in women who use estrogen-containing oral contraceptives[56].

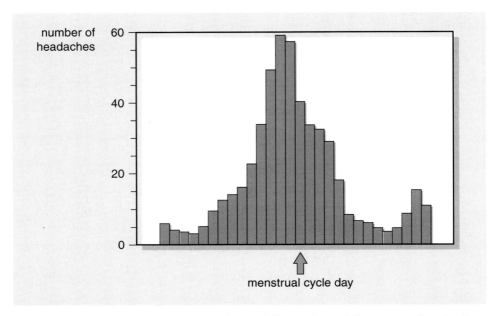

Figure 7.5. Frequency of headaches during different days of the menstrual cycle. Data represent 512 headaches recorded by 52 women who complained of premenstrual or menstrual migraine. The arrow denotes the first day of menstruation. Two-thirds of all headaches occurred within 4 days of the start of menstruation. Redrawn from reference 50

Pregnancy is associated with high levels of estrogen and progesterone. Some women experience their first migraine attack while pregnant[57]. More typically, however, migraineurs experience a reduction in headache frequency during pregnancy[57,58], especially women with a history of premenstrual or menstrual migraine[59]. For such women, headaches may then recur in the puerperium[60].

The prevalence of migraine is highest between ages 35 and 45 years[43]. Although migraine frequency declines with age[43,51], the menopause *per se* has little effect on migraine[61]. Effects of estrogen replacement therapy on migraine symptoms are variable, and hormone replacement occasionally contributes to migraine symptoms[56].

MULTIPLE SCLEROSIS

Multiple sclerosis is a common, chronic disorder of central nervous system white matter. Disease is thought to represent an autoimmune process mediated primarily

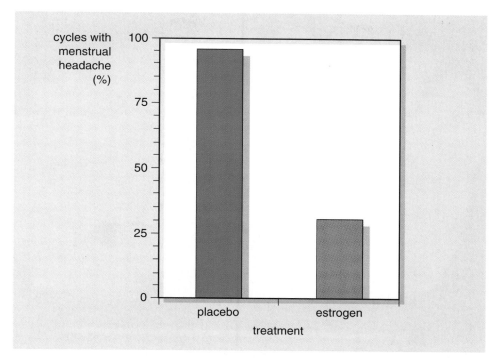

Figure 7.6. Effect of estrogen in reducing premenstrual or menstrual migraine headache. Eighteen women with menstrual migraine were treated with transcutaneous estradiol (1.5 mg/day for 7 days) or placebo in a double-blind cross-over trial conducted over the course of three consecutive menstrual cycles. As indicated in the figure, estrogen significantly reduced the number of menstrual cycles in which a headache occurred. Moreover, attacks that occurred during estrogen treatment were milder in intensity and shorter in duration than those that occurred during placebo treatment. Data are from reference 54

by T-cell lymphocytes and directed against specific myelin antigens. Myelin is produced by oligodendrocytes, and axons invaginated within the myelin sheath are secondarily damaged by the inflammatory response. Confluent areas of demyelination within the brain are referred to as plaques (Figure 7.7).

A patient's particular neurological deficits depend on the focal distribution of plaques, which can be found in the cerebrum, cerebellum, brain stem, spinal cord and optic nerves[62]. Symptoms are typically episodic, waxing and waning over a course of many years. Acute exacerbations are followed by residual deficits that accumulate with time. For some, the course is unremitting. Onset is often in

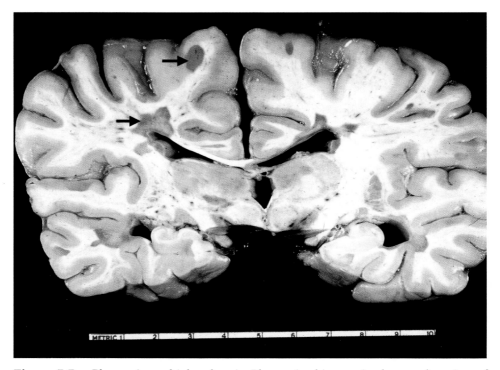

Figure 7.7. Plaques in multiple sclerosis. Plaques in this unstained coronal section of brain appear as dark lesions. Two plaques are indicated by arrows. Reproduced with permission from reference 62

young adulthood but can occur later. Like other illnesses thought to have an autoimmune pathogenesis[63], multiple sclerosis affects women more often than men.

Estrogens possess anti–inflammatory properties. Estrogen interacts with the hypothalamus, pituitary gland, ovaries and thymus gland to influence both humoral and cell-mediated immunity[64]. Estrogen actions include inhibition of leukocyte production in the bone marrow, suppression of delayed hypersensitivity, enhancement of antibody production and modulation of cytokine production by T–cell lymphocytes[65–68].

The clinical relevance of estrogen in multiple sclerosis is poorly established. Women who have used oral contraceptives are not at increased risk for multiple sclerosis[69]. Neurological relapses are reduced during pregnancy but increased in the postpartum period[70–75] (Figure 7.8), an effect also noted for certain other

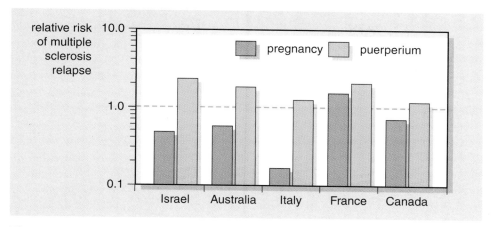

Figure 7.8. Relapse rate of multiple sclerosis during pregnancy and the puerperium. Case–control and cohort studies from five different countries indicate that the risk of neurological relapse is less during pregnancy than during the first 6 months postpartum. Data are from reference 70 (Israel), reference 71 (Australia), reference 72 (Italy), reference 73 (France) and reference 74 (Canada), as summarized in reference 75

autoimmune illnesses. Pregnancy does not appear to have a deleterious effect on long-term disability in this illness, nor is disability increased by multiple pregnancies[76]. Effects of menopause or of postmenopausal hormone therapy on neurological symptoms and on the long-term course of multiple sclerosis are unknown.

REFERENCES

1. Pfaff D, Keiner M. Atlas of estradiol-concentrating cells in the central nervous system of the female rat. *J Comp Neurol* 1973;151:121–58
2. Roy EJ, Buyer DR, Licari VA. Estradiol in the striatum: effects on behavior and dopamine receptors but no evidence for membrane steroid receptors. *Brain Res Bull* 1990;25:221–7
3. Joseph JA, Kochman K, Roth GS. Reduction of motor behavioural deficits in senescence via chronic prolactin or estrogen administration: time course and putative mechanisms of action. *Brain Res* 1989;505:195–202
4. Chiodo LA, Caggiula AR. Alterations in basal firing rate and autoreceptor sensitivity of dopamine neurons in the substantia nigra following acute and extended exposure to estrogen. *Eur J Pharmacol* 1980;67:165–6
5. Hruska RE, Silbergeld EK. Increased dopamine receptor sensitivity after estrogen treatment using the rat rotation model. *Science* 1980;208:1466–8
6. Willson P, Preece AA. Chorea gravidarum. *Arch Intern Med* 1932;49:471–533, 671–97
7. Lewis BV, Parsons M. Chorea gravidarum. *Lancet* 1966;1:284–6

8. Nausieda PA, Koller WC, Weiner WJ, Klawans HL. Chorea induced by oral contraceptives. *Neurology* 1979;29:1605–9

9. Quinn NP, Marsden CD. Menstrual-related fluctuations in Parkinson's disease. *Movement Dis* 1986;1:85–7

10. Gratton L. Neuroleptiques, parkinsonnisme et schizophrénie. *Union Med Canada* 1960;89: 679–94

11. Bedard P, Langelier P, Villeneuve A. Oestrogens and extrapyramidal system [Letter]. *Lancet* 1977;2:1367–8

12. Koller WC, Barr A, Biary N. Estrogen treatment of dyskinetic disorders. *Neurology* 1982; 32:547–9

13. Villeneuve A, Cazejust T, Côté M. Estrogens in tardive dyskinesia in male psychiatric patients. *Neuropsychobiology* 1980;6:145–51

14. Dluzen DE, McDermott JL, Liu B. Estrogen as a neuroprotectant against MPTP-induced neurotoxicity in C57/B1 mice. *Neurotoxicol Teratol* 1996;18:603–6

15. Marder K, Tang M-X, Alfaro B, *et al.* Postmenopausal estrogen use and Parkinson's disease with and without dementia. *Neurology* 1998;50:1141–3

16. Clark CM, Ewbank D, Lerner A, *et al.* The relationship between extrapyramidal signs and cognitive performance in patients with Alzheimer's disease enrolled in the CERAD study. *Neurology* 1997;49:70–5

17. Hansen LA, Samuel W. Criteria for Alzheimer's disease and the nosology of dementia with Lewy bodies. *Neurology* 1997;48:126–32

18. Logothetis J, Harner R. Electrocortical activation by estrogens. *Arch Neurol* 1960;3:290–7

19. Woolley DE, Timiras PS. The gonad–brain relationship: effects of female sex hormones on electroshock convulsions in the rat. *Endocrinology* 1962;70:196–209

20. Nicoletti F, Speciale C, Sortino MA, *et al.* Comparative effects of estradiol benzoate, the antiestrogen clomiphen citrate, and the progestin medroxyprogesterone acetate on kainic acid-induced seizures in male and female rats. *Epilepsia* 1985;26:252–7

21. Buterbaugh GG, Hudson GM. Estradiol replacement to female rats facilitates dorsal hippocampal but not ventral hippocampal kindled seizure acquisition. *Exp Neurol* 1991;111: 55–64

22. Terasawa E, Timiras PS. Electrical activity during the estrous cycle of the rat: cyclic changes in limbic structures. *Endocrinology* 1968;83:207–16

23. Kawakami M, Terasawa E, Ibuki T. Changes in multiple unit activity in the brain during the estrous cycle. *Neuroendocrinology* 1970;6:30–48

24. Wong M, Moss RL. Long-term and short-term electrophysiological effects of estrogen on the synaptic properties of hippocampal CA1 neurons. *J Neurosci* 1992;12:3217–25

25. Warren SG, Humphreys AG, Juraska JM, Greenough WT. LTP varies across the estrous cycle: enhanced synaptic plasticity in proestrus rats. *Brain Res* 1995;703:26–30

26. Woolley CS, McEwen BS. Estradiol mediates fluctuation in hippocampal synapse density during the estrous cycle in the adult rat. *J Neurosci* 1992;12:2549–54

27. Murphy DD, Segal M. Regulation of dendritic spine density in cultured rat hippocampal neurons by steroid hormones. *J Neurosci* 1996;16:4059–68

28. Logothetis J, Harner R, Morrell F, Torres T. The role of estrogens in catamenial exacerbation of epilepsy. *Neurology* 1959;9:352–60

29. Creutzfeldt OD, Arnold P-M, Becker D, *et al*. EEG changes during spontaneous and controlled menstrual cycles and their correlation with psychological performance. *Electroenceph Clin Neurophysiol* 1976;40:113–31

30. Dickerson WW. The effect of menstruation on seizure incidence. *J Nerv Ment Dis* 1941;94:160–9

31. Laidlaw J. Catamenial epilepsy. *Lancet* 1956;2:1235–7

32. Bäckström T. Epileptic seizures in women related to plasma estrogen and progesterone during the menstrual cycle. *Acta Neurol Scand* 1976;54:321–47

33. Rosciszewska D, Buntner B, Guz I, Zawisza L. Ovarian hormones, anticonvulsant drugs, and seizures during the menstrual cycle in women with epilepsy. *J Neurol Neurosurg Psychiatry* 1986;49:47–51

34. Donaldson JO. *Neurology of Pregnancy*, 2nd edn. Philadelphia: WB Saunders, 1989

35. Knight AH, Rhind EG. Epilepsy and pregnancy: a study of 153 pregnancies in 59 patients. *Epilepsia* 1975;16:99–110

36. Landgren S, Bäckström T, Kalistratov G. The effect of progesterone on the spontaneous interictal spike evoked by the application of penicillin to the cat's cerebral cortex. *J Neurol Sci* 1978;36:119–33

37. Mattson RH, Cramer JA, Caldwell BV, Siconolfi BC. Treatment of seizures with medroxyprogesterone acetate: preliminary report. *Neurology* 1984;34:1255–8

38. Herzog AG. Intermittent progesterone therapy and frequency of complex partial seizures in women with menstrual disorders. *Neurology* 1986;36:1607–10

39. Mattson RH, Cramer JA, Darney PD, Naftolin F. Use of oral contraceptives by women with epilepsy. *J Am Med Assoc* 1986;256:238–40

40. Lauritzen M, Olesen J. Regional cerebral blood flow during migraine attacks by xenon-133 inhalation and emission tomography. *Brain* 1984;107:447–61

41. Olesen J, Friberg L, Olsen TS, *et al*. Timing and topography of cerebral blood flow, aura, and headache during migraine attacks. *Ann Neurol* 1990;28:791–8

42. Woods RP, Iacoboni M, Mazziotta JC. Bilateral spreading cerebral hypoperfusion during spontaneous migraine headache. *N Engl J Med* 1994;331:1689–92

43. Stewart WF, Lipton RB, Celentano DD, Reed ML. Prevalence of migraine headache in the United States. *J Am Med Assoc* 1992;267:64–9

44. Belfort MA, Saade GR, Snabes M, *et al*. Hormonal status affects the reactivity of the cerebral vasculature. *Am J Obstet Gynecol* 1995;172:1273–8

45. Ohkura T, Teshima Y, Isse K, *et al*. Estrogen increases cerebral and cerebellar blood flows in postmenopausal women. *Menopause* 1995;2:13–18

46. Cohen IR, Wise PM. Effects of estradiol on the diurnal rhythm of serotonin activity in microdissected brain areas of ovariectomized rats. *Endocrinology* 1988;122:2619–25

47. Biegon A, Reches A, Snyder L, McEwen BS. Serotonergic and noradrenergic receptors in the rat brain: modulation by chronic exposure to ovarian hormones. *Life Sci* 1983;32:2015–21

48. Sumner BEH, Fink G. Estrogen increases the density of 5-hydroxytryptamine$_{2A}$ receptors in cerebral cortex and nucleus accumbens in the female rat. *J Steroid Biochem Mol Biol* 1995;54:15–20

49. Somerville BW. The role of estradiol withdrawal in the etiology of menstrual migraine. *Neurology* 1972;22:355–65

50. Dalton K. Progesterone suppositories and pessaries in the treatment of menstrual migraine. *Headache* 1973;12:151–9

51. Waters WE, O'Connor PJ. Epidemiology of headache and migraine in women. *J Neurol Neurosurg Psychiatry* 1971;34:148–53

52. Whitty CWM, Hockaday JM, Whitty MM. The effect of oral contraceptives on migraine. *Lancet* 1966;1:856–9

53. Magos A, Zilkha KJ, Studd JWW. Treatment of menstrual migraine by oestradiol implants. *J Neurol Neurosurg Psychiatry* 1983;46:1044–6

54. de Lignières B, Vincens M, Mauvais-Jarvis P, Mas JL, Touboul PJ, Bousser MG. Prevention of menstrual migraine by percutaneous oestradiol. *Br Med J* 1986;293:1540

55. Sarrel PM. Ovarian hormones and the circulation. *Maturitas* 1990;12:287–98

56. Kudrow L. The relationship of headache frequency to hormone use in migraine. *Headache* 1975;15:36–40

57. Somerville BW. A study of migraine in pregnancy. *Neurology* 1972;22:824–8

58. Chen T-C, Leviton A. Headache recurrence in pregnant women with migraine. *Headache* 1994;34:107–10

59. Lance JW, Anthony M. Some clinical aspects of migraine: a prospective study of 500 patients. *Arch Neurol* 1966;15:356–61

60. Stein GS. Headaches in the first post partum week and their relationship to migraine. *Headache* 1981;21:201–5

61. Whitty CWM, Hockaday JM. Migraine: a follow-up study of 92 patients. *Br Med J* 1968;1:735–6

62. Poser CM. *An Atlas of Multiple Sclerosis*. Carnforth, UK: Parthenon Publishing, 1998

63. Martin R, McFarland HF. Immunological aspects of experimental allergic encephalo-myelitis and multiple sclerosis. *Crit Rev Clin Lab Sci* 1995;32:121–82

64. Grossman CJ. Interactions between the gonadal steroids and the immune sytstem. *Science* 1985;227:257–61

65. Gilmore W, Weiner LP, Correale J. Effect of estradiol on cytokine secretion by proteolipid protein-specific T cell clones isolated from multiple sclerosis patients and normal control subjects. *J Immunol* 1997;158:446–51

66. Josefsson E, Tarkowski A, Carlsten H. Anti-inflammatory properties of estrogen. *Cell Immunol* 1992;142:67–78

67. Carlsten H, Holmdahl R, Tarkowski A, Nilsson L-A. Oestradiol- and testosterone-mediated effects on the immune system in normal and autoimmune mice are genetically linked and inherited as dominant traits. *Immunology* 1989;68:209–14

68. Pacifici R, Brown C, Puscheck E, *et al.* Effect of surgical menopause and estrogen replacement on cytokine release from human blood mononuclear cells. *Proc Natl Acad Sci USA* 1991;88:5134–8

69. Villard-Mackintosk L, Vessey MP. Oral contraceptives and reproductive factors in multiple sclerosis incidence. *Contraception* 1993;47:161–8

70. Korn-Lubetzki I, Kahana E, Cooper G, Abramsky O. Activity of multiple sclerosis during pregnancy and puerperium. *Ann Neurol* 1984;16:229–31

71. Frith JA, McLeod JG. Pregnancy and multiple sclerosis. *J Neurol Neurosurg Psychiatry* 1988;51:495–8

72. Bernardi S, Grasso MG, Bertollini R, Orzi F, Fieschi C. The influence of pregnancy on relapses in multiple sclerosis: a cohort study. *Acta Neurol Scand* 1991;84:403–6

73. Roullet E, Verdier-Taillefer MH, Amarenco P, Gharbi G, Alperovitch A, Marteau R. Pregnancy and multiple sclerosis: a longitudinal study of 125 remittent patients. *J Neurol Neurosurg Psychiatry* 1993;56:1062–5

74. Sadovnick AD, Eisen K, Hashimoto SA, *et al*. Pregnancy and multiple sclerosis: a prospective study. *Arch Neurol* 1994;51:1120–4

75. Damek DM, Shuster EA. Pregnancy and multiple sclerosis. *Mayo Clin Proc* 1997;72:977–89

76. Thompson DS, Nelson LM, Burns A, Burks JS, Franklin GM. The effects of pregnancy in multiple sclerosis: a retrospective study. *Neurology* 1986;36:1097–9

8
Future directions

Worldwide, almost half a billion women are postmenopausal[1]. For many of these women, issues surrounding the use of hormone therapy are immediate and pressing. Recent research results confirm that estrogen affects central nervous system functioning directly and indirectly, in manners both widely distributed and discrete. Clinical findings adumbrate meaningful benefits for mood and cognition, and suggest influences on several neurological disorders. Nevertheless, many clinical implications of hormone therapy remain unsettled. Human observational data are not always coherent, and convincing data from randomized controlled trials are still exiguous. With respect to cognition, for example, cogent literature analyses argue both for and against a convincing benefit of estrogen[2,3].

No questions of hormone therapy and the brain are more important than those that deal with dementia. If epidemiological projections prove correct[2,4], the widespread use of postmenopausal estrogen could reduce by more than one million the number of women in the United States with Alzheimer's disease. Thus far, however, human data are observational, and clinical guidelines on dementia prevention are not anchored by findings from double-blind controlled trials. Several randomized trials are now under way, however. In the United States, the best known of these involves older women enrolled in a large government-sponsored study known as the Women's Health Initiative. Over 7500 healthy women randomized to receive conjugated estrogens (with or without a progestogen, depending on the presence or absence of a uterus) are being monitored for endpoints that include an Alzheimer's diagnosis[5]. Results of this potentially epochal study are not anticipated until about the year 2006. Other studies are underway in the United Kingdom and elsewhere.

For some neurophysiological processes, estrogen effects can be accentuated or opposed by progesterone[6,7]. Because long-term unopposed estrogen therapy puts women with a uterus at risk for endometrial cancer[8], estrogen replacement almost always includes a progestogen. For women with a uterus, parallel studies would be needed to verify that continuous or sequential treatment with a progestogen does not detract from anticipated estrogen benefits. For example, concerns that a progestogen might impact on coronary heart disease unfavorably necessitated an intervention trial that compared the effects of both unopposed and opposed estrogens on serum lipoproteins, lipids and other coronary risk factors[9]. In a neurological sphere, clinical findings imply that progestogens may adversely impact mood, feelings of well-being and possibly even cognition[10-12], or that progestogens could attenuate putative beneficial effects of estrogen on Alzheimer's symptoms[13]. Each clinical condition will need to be separately considered, however.

If clinical trials indicate that estrogen, with or without a progestogen, has a clinically meaningful role in mood and cognition, or in cerebrovascular disease and other specific neurological disorders, then new studies will be needed to confirm precise mechanisms by which beneficial effects are realized. Understanding the mechanisms of action would facilitate the identification and development of estrogenic compounds that maximize clinical benefit or the utilization of non-estrogenic compounds that work more effectively via similar presumptive pathways. The recognition that receptor-mediated actions of estrogen may be tissue-selective implies the exciting possibility that unintended neurological or systemic side-effects could be minimized without sacrificing the desirable effects on target symptoms.

REFERENCES

1. Hill K. The demography of menopause. *Maturitas* 1996;23:113–27
2. Yaffe K, Sawaya G, Lieberburg I, Grady D. Estrogen therapy in postmenopausal women. *J Am Med Assoc* 1998;279:688–95
3. Haskell SG, Richardson ED, Horwitz RI. The effect of estrogen replacement therapy on cognitive function in women: a critical review of the literature. *J Clin Epidemiol* 1997;50:1249–64
4. Henderson VW. The epidemiology of estrogen replacement therapy and Alzheimer's disease. *Neurology* 1997;48(Suppl 7):27–35
5. Shumaker SA, Reboussin BA, Espeland MA, *et al.* The Women's Health Initiative Memory Study (WHIMS): a trial of the effect of estrogen therapy in preventing and slowing the progression of dementia. *Controlled Clin Trials* 1998;19:604–21
6. Woolley CS, McEwen BS. Roles of estradiol and progesterone in regulation of hippocampal dendritic spine density during the estrous cycle in the rat. *J Comp Neurol* 1993;336:293–306
7. Gibbs RB. Fluctuations in relative levels of choline acetyltransferase mRNA in different regions of the rat basal forebrain across the estrus cycle: effects of estrogen and progestrone. *J Neurosci* 1996;16:1049–55

8. Weiss NS, Hill DA. Postmenopausal estrogens and progestogens and the incidence of gynecologic cancer. *Maturitas* 1996;23:235–9

9. Writing group for the PEPI trial. Effects of estrogen or estrogen/progestin regimens on heart disease risk factors in postmenopausal women: the postmenopausal estrogen/ progestin interventions (PEPI) trial. *J Am Med Assoc* 1995;273:199–208

10. Sherwin BB. The impact of different doses of estrogen and progestin on mood and sexual behavior in postmenopausal women. *J Clin Endocrinol Metab* 1991;72:336–43

11. Freeman EW, Purdy RH, Coutifaris C, Rickels K, Paul SM. Anxiolytic metabolites of progesterone: correlation with mood and performance measures following oral progesterone administration to healthy female volunteers. *Neuroendocrinology* 1993;58:478–84

12. Zweifel JE, O'Brien WH. A meta-analysis of the effect of hormone replacement therapy upon depressed mood. *Psychoneuroendocrinology* 1997;22:189–212

13. Ohkura T, Isse K, Akazawa K, Hamamoto M, Yaoi Y, Hagino N. Long-term estrogen replacement therapy in female patients with dementia of the Alzheimer type: 7 case reports. *Dementia* 1995;6:99–107

Index

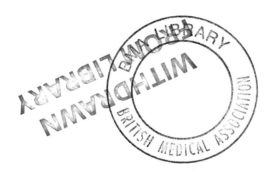